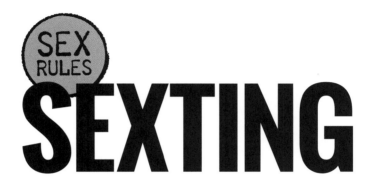

SEXTING

THE GROWNUP'S LITTLE BOOK OF SEX TIPS FOR GETTING DIRTY DIGITALLY

TINA HORN

FAIR WINDS

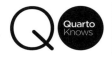

Quarto is the authority on a wide range of topics.

Quarto educates, entertains and enriches the lives of
our readers—enthusiasts and lovers of hands-on living.

www.QuartoKnows.com

© 2016 Quarto Publishing Group USA Inc.

First published in the USA in 2016 by
Fair Winds Press, an imprint of
Quarto Publishing Group USA Inc.
100 Cummings Center
Suite 406-L
Beverly, MA 01915-6101
QuartoKnows.com
Visit our blogs at QuartoKnows.com

20 19 18 17 16   1 2 3 4 5

ISBN: 978-1-59233-705-7

Digital edition published in 2016
eISBN: 978-1-62788-827-1

Library of Congress Cataloging-in-Publication Data available

Cover, book, and illustration design by Mattie Wells: mattiewells.com

Printed and bound in China

For Andie Lynn: In honor of all the
ways we're different that show us
all the ways we're the same

CONTENTS

USE YOUR WORDS:

PUT YOURSELF OUT THERE:

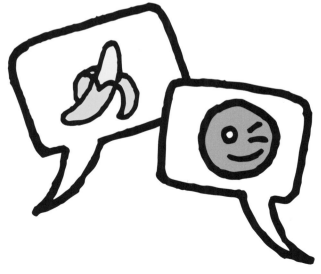

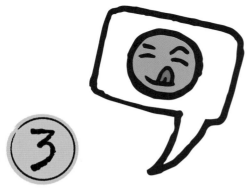

3

DISCOVER THE JOYS OF SEXT:

USING TECHNOLOGY TO STAY TURNED ON

4

SEND SEXY PICTURES AND VIDEO:

A SELFIE SAYS A THOUSAND (DIRTY) WORDS

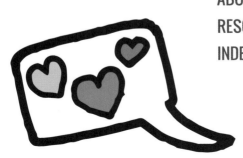

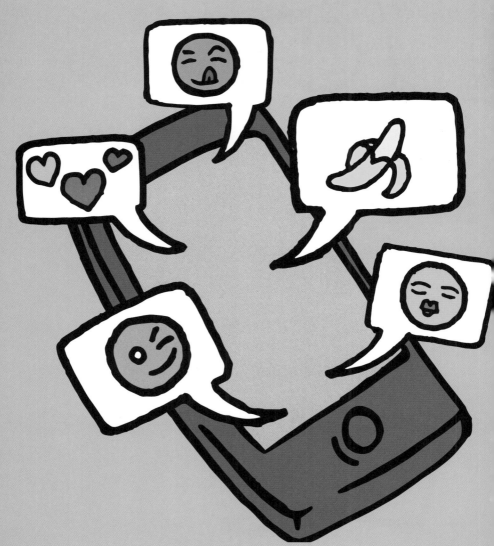

"I WANT YOU." Is there anything sexier than hearing those three little words spoken by someone who you want right back?

"I want you to come home with me," says your date, leaning across the restaurant table to give you an electric touch on your thigh.

*

Your phone lights up with a message:

I want you inside me tonight.

*

Your partner's face fills up your computer screen and stares deep into your eyes. When he speaks, you feel like he is whispering in your ear, even though he is hundreds of miles away. He says,

I need to rip your clothes off.

I'm so fucking horny for you.

I have designs on your body.

Whether you're in the same room or mediated by a computer, this kind of fantastic dirty talk has the power to turn you on, get you off, and bring you and your partner closer together.

For almost ten years, it's been my job to communicate about sex. I've coached private clients about their kinky fantasies and directed hardcore indie porn. I've published queer erotica, written nonfiction articles on sexual subcultures, and spoken to lecture halls filled with curious students. On my podcast, *Why Are People Into That?!*, my guests and I chat explicitly about everything from exhibitionism to spanking to anal play.

For me, sex and verbal communication are inextricably intertwined. Language brings us together. Words create romantic poetry and essential boundaries, defusing conflict and promoting understanding. Dirty talk is a powerful tool and an exciting toy for generating attraction and connection

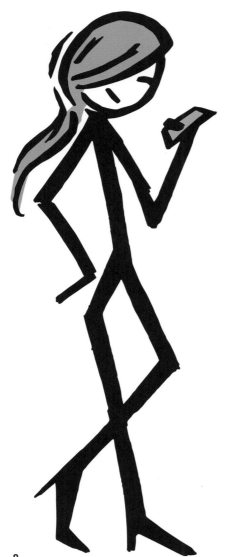

between people. Sometimes the best kind of language is wordless: it exists in a glance, a pose, or a perfectly composed image.

Communicating in our modern digital world—a culture of computers, devices, apps, and cameras—can be overwhelming. New methods for exchanging virtual messages seem to crop up every week. In this age, you can hit the dating world after a few short years of a monogamous relationship only to feel like everyone is fluent in a dialect you didn't even know existed. However, the point of technology is to bring us together, not tear us apart. We need to make each new development work for us, rather than leave us behind.

With the communication skills you'll learn from this book, you'll develop the confidence to have the kind of sex you want to have and connect with the people you want to have it with. You'll learn to think of dirty talk as a sex toy for that big organ between your ears! You'll also learn how to use your personal computer to become a veritable erotic filmmaker and superstar, albeit one who is creating a private collection with an exclusive audience.

In chapter 1, we'll cover the basics of dirty talk, from learning your favorite vocabulary words to exploring role-play fantasies. Chapter 2 will teach you to navigate the evolving world of hookup apps and dating sites. Everything you've ever wanted to know about digital flirting and the syntax of sexting is in chapter 3. A naked picture says a thousand words in chapter 4, where you'll learn how to take flattering selfies that stay secure.

This book is for anyone who wants to deepen his or her sexual communication. I'm a queer cisgender woman who is partnered and nonmonogamous. I don't make any assumptions about your gender or the gender of the person or persons you sleep with. In my writing, I'm inclined to switch gender pronouns around, and I trust you to make adjustments accordingly.

Dirty talk and private show-off pics can be a way to reclaim words that make us feel fabulous about our bodies and relationships. They can also help us assert our identities and explore our fantasies. Excellent erotic communication is about cursing a blue streak in bed. It's about creating a teasing video just for your partner, or sending him or her a detailed description of what you want to do tonight. Most important, though, it's about asserting what you want and listening to what your partners want so you can make each other happy and fulfilled.

I'm looking forward to making cunning linguists of you all!

1

USE YOUR WORDS:
The Basics of Dirty Talk

Before you send your first sext, before you agonize over your OkCupid survey answers, before you take the perfect butt selfie, you have to know the basics of dirty talking "IRL." (That's "in real life" in Internet speak— you know, that place where you're in the same room as another person, where you can smell and touch them in three dimensions!)

My most popular workshops over the years have always been the ones that focus on sexual communication. When I ask my students why they signed up for that particular class, by far the most common reason is:

"I just don't know what to say."

Do you find yourself frozen with stage fright mid-seduction, like an actress who has forgotten her lines? Do your partners encourage you to use nasty words while you're having sex, and yet you have no clue what would turn them on?

Maybe you find yourself stuttering because the blood is rushing *away* from your brain. Perhaps, like many of us, you were so socialized to think of sex as an impolite conversation topic that you're scared to talk about it even while you're actually doing it.

I honestly believe that people *do* know what to say; they just need a little help with *how* to say it. You are the person who knows what you want. You have the right to ask for it. This section is going to give you all the tricks you'll need to feel confident about expressing your inner desires in the heat of the moment.

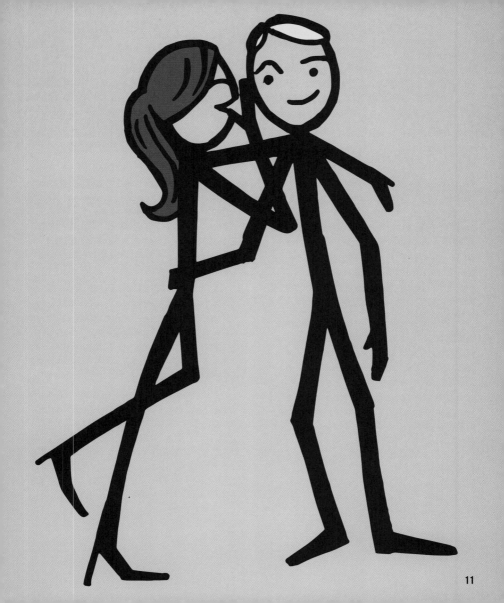

Perhaps what you want is a long, deep kiss. Or maybe you want to be naked and sweaty, lustfully tearing one another apart. You could have a special fetish you're not sure how to ask for. You may need romance, intimacy, or commitment. Regardless, you're only going to get what you're after if you know how to ask for it.

DON'T WORRY ABOUT BEING SILLY

Why does sex make us feel ridiculous sometimes? Perhaps it's because our sexual nature can feel distinct, messier, and more primal than our everyday selves. Letting go completely can be so terrifying. We don't say the things we really want to say to our partners because we think if we stay quiet we can protect our vulnerable feelings.

I am here to tell you that you will have the best sex possible when you abandon yourself to pleasure. A strange thing happens when you're aroused and in the moment with your partner: all logic and rationality shift. You can behave like a pampered princess when in real life you're a strong-willed lady. You can

call your partner a word in the bedroom that you would never call him at a dinner party. The sillier you allow yourself to be, the more fun you'll have. The best sex partner will be more turned on by you the more you let yourself go, and that includes running your mouth off.

This book is filled with sentences and words that are going to make you giggle when you first read them and say them out loud. In addition to laughter, these words have the power to bring you the hardest orgasms and the deepest connections you've ever experienced.

Let's start with some classic catchphrases, so you can get in touch with your inner porn star.

PRACTICE MAKES PERFECT

Dirty talk is as much about saying things that make *you* feel sexy as it is about knowing what your partner wants to hear. That's why I recommend starting solo, to learn more about your own desires.

Choose one of the sentences from below, and practice saying it passionately over and over again until it sounds natural, until you're used to the sound of your voice saying it. Say it to yourself in the mirror. Say it to yourself while you masturbate! (If you don't already have a healthy solo sex routine, I recommend it very highly for self-knowledge, self-confidence, and stress relief!)

TINA'S TIPS:
TOP TEN SENTENCES TO PRACTICE
(Use kissing as an example, but any activity will work.)

I love the way you kiss me.

The way you kiss me feels so good.

Please may I kiss you?

It really turns me on when you kiss me like that.

Yeah, you like it when I kiss you, don't you?

Don't ever stop kissing me!

You look so good when you're kissing me.

Do you want me to keep kissing you?

You are the best kisser in the entire world.

I need you to kiss me right now!

PRIVATE DIRTY NOTEBOOK

This may sound old-fashioned in a book about sexting, but you should get yourself a notebook. It could be a cheap composition book or a fancy, leather-bound Moleskine. Remember, this is like your diary with the heart-shaped lock, or your personal captain's log, meant for your eyes only. Label it as top secret and keep it in a safe space so that you can feel free to express your true sexual self.

Create a yes/no/maybe list. What sexy things do you love, what is definitely off-limits, and what are you curious about trying?

Keep track of your sex dreams. Write them down just after you've woken up, before they start to fade away.

Try the same thing with your masturbation fantasies. Let your mind wander and then record what you think about it in your most honest private moments of arousal.

Write original erotica. Your stories don't have to be highly literary! Just compose a filthy description of something you'd like to have happen, however implausible.

Copy down your favorite sexts. Back when I had a flip-phone with limited space, I would copy down my best texts longhand before deleting them. I found I always remembered those phrases most vividly! You could also take a screenshot and save it in a private folder called "best sexts."

Try an automatic writing exercise. Set a timer for ten minutes. Write everything you can think about your ideal online hook-up, one-night-stand, threesome, kinky adventure, romantic vacation, or any other scenario you want. Don't consider anybody else's needs; see what happens when you're selfish!

Make lists. Your favorite sex acts, sex partners, sex scenes from movies, celebrities you'd like to bone, and co-workers you daydream about are just a few examples.

Watch some porn and write a review. What did you like and not like? What would you like to try?

Read some erotica and write a book report. Which parts turned you on, and why?

Read parts of your notebook aloud. Record it and listen back to yourself.

GETTING WHAT YOU WANT

Now that you have some sentences in your repertoire, it's time to start using them with other humans to make your hot sex even hotter.

Let's say you're out on a fun date with someone awesome and you have decided you'd like to sleep with her. Strategize what you want your date to know about your sexuality. Mention that your favorite part of the television show *Scandal* is all the steamy sex scenes. Bring up an article from the *New York Times* about the search for female Viagra. Mention your favorite polyamory podcast or a local play party you've heard about. If you can discuss sexuality in a general way, you can learn a lot about one another without the pressure of discussing what is hopefully about to go down between the two of you!

The crucial thing to keep in mind is that you have the right to assert what you like, what you lust for, and what you're in the mood for. Of course, you also want to know the same thing about your date, so be a good listener!

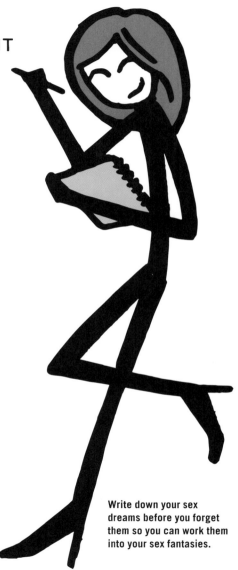

Write down your sex dreams before you forget them so you can work them into your sex fantasies.

EROTIC NEGOTIATION

One of the first things I learned when I started experimenting with bondage, spanking, and other kinds of BDSM was the importance of "kink negotiation." Before incorporating erotic pain or restraint into sex, it was crucial that my partner and I discussed consent, limits, safe words, and pervy desires. It was sort of like consulting a recipe book before cooking an elaborate dinner to make sure we didn't burn the kitchen to the ground!

Honestly, whether you're playing with whips and chains or enjoying the vanilla side, all sexy times could do with a little negotiation. The more you can clarify beforehand, the more you can let yourself go and experience the moment you're about to have.

Imagine you're making out in the cab on the way back to your place. Now would be a great time to start the kind of conversation that is best had with your clothes on, when you can think straight.

Whisper one of the following sentences in your date's ear:

What do you want to do with me when we get to my room?

I can't wait to get you in my bed so I can put your mouth to work.

Are you excited to see me with my clothes off?

If we weren't in this cab I would already be sucking your cock by now.

This is also the ideal moment to have a conversation about birth control, STI status, and monogamy parameters. Many people find these kinds of conversations awkward, but they can actually be responsible and titillating at the same time.

I can't wait to fuck you. Do you have condoms at your place or should we stop at the store first?

Hey, I just want you to know I'm sleeping with a few other people right now. I'm having lots of fun with you and would love for you to be one of them.

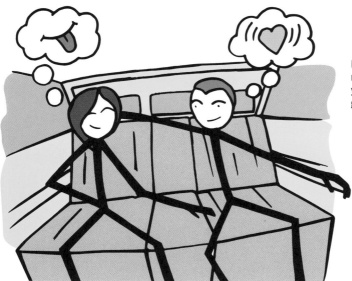

Hold erotic negotiations before you and your date get down and dirty.

TINA'S TIPS:

HOW TO NOT BE A SLUT SHAMER

"Slut shaming" is a term to describe any judgment made toward someone for having lots of partners, being voraciously insatiable, or just simply loving sex. Women tend to experience disproportional amounts of slut shaming because of the double standards many cultures share about the sexual worth of different genders.

Slut shamers are merely revealing their own insecurities and fears. Unfortunately, many people become shy about expressing their needs because they have been stifled in the past.

When someone tells you which words, styles, activities, or fetishes they love, make sure to remember they are making themselves vulnerable to you. Try to be affirming, even if what they like is not exactly your thing.

A LITTLE TO THE LEFT . . .

So how can you use language to get what you want once you're alone together? Well, dirty talk is not only good for seduction, it's also great for guidance, encouragement, and stimulation.

Sometimes we don't want to give direction to our lovers because we're worried we'll sound like we're nagging. Let's say you're happy with what's happening, but you'd like to make an adjustment. Say your date is playing with your G-spot, but she's going way too hard, and you'd like her to go down on you for a while instead. Let's make a distinction between constructive guidance and directions that cause someone to feel shut down.

When you say, "I don't like that," you're creating a dead end for your partner. Instead, try redirecting her to a different road you want her to drive! One way to deflect attention away from something you're not in the mood for is to begin to talk dirty about something else entirely:

I want you to go down on me so badly right now.

I want you to put that sweet mouth to work.

I need to fuck your face immediately.

I bet fucking me is making you really horny.

Please, can I touch you?

I love what you're doing, could you do it a little slower, babe?

Mmm, you're so good with your hands, it makes me want your cock inside me.

TINA'S TIPS:
THE COMPLIMENT SANDWICH

I really don't enjoy it when a play partner pinches my nipples. However, I do love having my breasts played with roughly, or having my nipples teased softly. So when someone tweaks me, instead of reacting by saying, "Ouch!" or "Don't do that, I hate that!" I have a few lines ready.

One strategy is giving a reason that has nothing to do with the person: "Oh, honey, my nipples are super sensitive, so it really turns me on when you're gentle with them."

Or I can give another, related suggestion: "You know what I really love? I love having my tits groped really hard, like this!" Then I demonstrate on myself, or maybe on my partner, how I like it done.

Social workers call this technique the Compliment Sandwich or the Feedback Sandwich. It's incredibly effective. The idea is to give constructive criticism wedged between two pieces of compliment bread:

I love this thing / Could you change this thing / You sexy thing!

When you accentuate the positive, it makes it a lot easier to discuss the ways things could be even better.

STAND UP FOR YOURSELF

When I encourage you to try not to shut your partner down in your sexual communication, I am *not* saying that you don't have the right to say no to something you don't want. On the contrary, it is extremely important to be able to firmly say *no* and to be heard and respected for that. If you don't want to have sex, or you don't want to have a certain kind of sex, you always have the right to speak up. When someone says *no* to you, it's essential that you listen, even if you find it confusing, hurtful, or disappointing.

Remember the "Yes/No/Maybe" list from your erotic notebook? It can be just as hard to stand up for things you *don't* want as it is to say what you *do* want.

Your boundaries and needs are as an integral part of your sex life as your desires are. Language is the most powerful way to establish consent, and no sexual encounter is complete without consent. Boundaries are not negative things: the parameters of your no's create a wonderful world of yeses for you and your partner to explore together.

FLATTERY WILL GET YOU EVERYWHERE

Everyone wants to feel beautiful, to feel like a sexual superhero. When I give my date a compliment, I'm showing that I can think about someone else. I also demonstrate that I can pay attention to detail and read body language, which is a signal that I'm good in the sack. I use compliments to put people at ease, to help them feel relaxed and receptive.

Compliment Givers

Try a compliment when you're in public, during your initial flirtation. Comment on something specific about your date's outfit. Pay attention to how he responds. Listen to the things he values. Does he love to talk about going to the gym? Run your hand along his forearm muscles and tell him you love how defined they are. And who doesn't like to be complimented on his hair?

Consider the role that gender plays in compliments. A masculine person may feel affirmed by being called handsome more than beautiful. If someone is petite, she is probably used to being called cute; try calling her gorgeous instead and see how she responds.

As you get to know people, you'll learn about their insecurities. This could be a good chance to show you love the parts of them they have trouble loving about themselves. For example, your curvy partner might like to be told she is *thick, juicy*, or *zaftig*. If you have a partner with a smaller-than-average penis that you think is the perfect size, tell him exactly that!

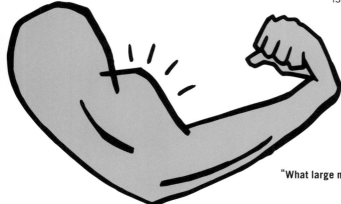

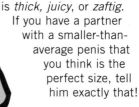

"What large muscles you have!"

21

Compliment Receivers

Think about a part of your body that you love people to notice. Are you proud of your long, luscious hair, your rock-hard abs, or your bubble butt? Ask for attention and worship on that part of your body, and show your appreciation when you get it.

When someone compliments you, be gracious. Women in particular are socialized to deflect flattery. We're told to put constant effort into our appearance but not to be proud of it. If someone says, "You look sexy tonight," don't say, "Oh, no, I must look a wreck, I'm so tired!" Instead, simply smile and say thank you!

X-Rated Flattery

Polite exchanges of flattery are great practice for the more X-rated versions.

Tell your date how sexy she looks without her clothes on. When she is doing something well, make sure you tell her so she keeps doing it!

You look so pretty with your face buried in my pussy.

Oh my god, you are so good at pounding me!

Your cock tastes so good! I have to have it in my mouth!

Nobody fucks my ass like you do!

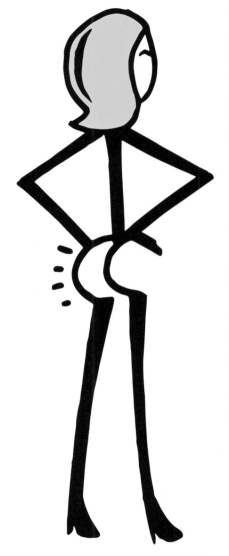

"How great does my ass look in these jeans?"

TINA'S TIPS:
BE REAL BE FABULOUS

In the summer of 2012, I was single and finally getting over my last big breakup. It was my first vacation from graduate school since I had moved to Brooklyn. I was ready to sample the all-you-can-eat buffet of this romantic, hot, slutty city.

This was when I made my first ever online dating account, on OkCupid. I did not have a smartphone at the time, so I could only check my messages when I settled down on my laptop with my apartment's janky Wi-Fi.

Every day when I got home, I checked my email, my personal Facebook, my professional social media streams, and my OkCupid messages. Toggling back and forth between windows kept me from getting too sucked in or obsessive with any one task.

At the time, my ideal person to find would have been an ongoing fuck buddy. Someone with whom I could enjoy some beers, duet to a Clash song at a karaoke bar, and then ride our bikes home for some sweaty, dirty sex. The message I put out on my profile was definitely cavalier: a "confident queer lady, loves spanking and rock 'n' roll, looking for fun" kinda vibe.

I had some fun times, and some confusing disappointments, and I definitely learned a lot about how OkCupid does and doesn't work for me. Right now, I'm not single or looking, but if I were to post a new profile today, I know I would approach it exactly the same way. I would be really real about everything I think makes me fabulous and only go out with people who could understand and appreciate me.

THE POWER OF SUGGESTION

You're locked in a passionate embrace. You want to make the most of it! You want the hardest orgasms, the screaming, the sweat, the endorphins, and the tangled sheets. This is the moment when language becomes more than seduction, more than consent: This is the moment when dirty talk becomes the sex toy that makes every orgasm harder. So where do you start?

Believe it or not, the trick to talking dirty in the sack all comes down to one word: narrate.

Imagine you're going down on your partner. He's hard and hot in your mouth, and you're working him up with every blowjob skill you've ever learned. You look up at him, he looks down at you, and he says:

You're sucking my cock.

This may sound absurd out of context. Put yourself in the moment, or better yet, add this dialogue to your masturbation fantasies. Remember our first rule about being silly? It can be so hot to acknowledge how absurd sex can be.

Think about how you might narrate other sex acts:

Oh my god you're fucking me.

I feel you deep in my ass.

I'm getting the spanking I deserve.

Now let's take it to the next level. Let's describe how arousing that blowjob is:

Your hot wet little mouth has me so hard for you right now.

Does sucking my dick make your pussy wet?

Holy shit, you're turning me on you little cocksucker.

Now let's combine flattery with our narration:

You are the best cocksucker in the entire world. This is the best blowjob of my life. You are so fucking good at that, baby.

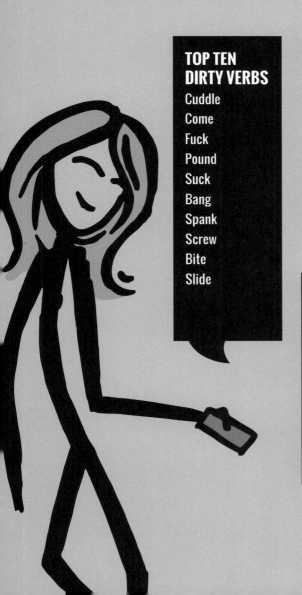

TOP TEN DIRTY VERBS
Cuddle
Come
Fuck
Pound
Suck
Bang
Spank
Screw
Bite
Slide

TOP TEN DESCRIPTIVE SEXY WORDS

Hard	Hairy
Wet	Hot
Red	Sweet
Strong	Tight
Smooth	Nasty

TOP TEN INSTRUCTIVE WORDS/PHRASES

Yes	Do it!
No	Now
Please	Slower/faster/harder/lighter
May I?	
Ma'am	Need
Sir	

25

LET'S GET PHYSICAL

There's a reason that many curse words refer to the most private parts of human anatomy. Vulgarity is a powerful tool that you can use for your own erotic purposes. Some people have filthy buzzwords that turn them on every single time, and those words are often R-rated terms for body parts. Use the following pages to discover the words you and your partner like for your body parts.

WORDS FOR WHAT YOU'VE GOT BETWEEN YOUR LEGS

Pussy   Snatch
Cunt   Dick
Hole   Prick
Cock   Junk
Clit

WORDS FOR FLUIDS

Cum
Jiz
Juice
Spunk
Sweat
Spit

WORDS FOR OTHER SEXY BODY PARTS

Hair   Feet
Hands   Hips
Fingers   Belly
Toes   Muscles

WORDS FOR SECONDARY SEXUAL CHARACTERISTICS

Mouth   Balls
Tits   Tongue
Nipples   Lips

WORDS FOR THE GREATEST BODY PART OF ALL TIME

Butt   Rump
Ass   Derrière
Asshole   Booty

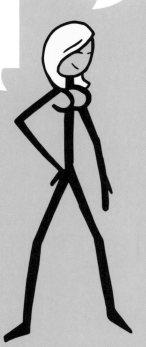
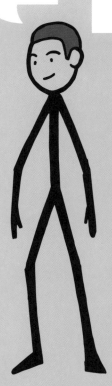

Use compliments and arousal words that turn you on and let your partner know how sexy you find him or her.

DIRTY TALK FILL-IN-THE-BLANKS

1. Compliment:
I really love the way you **verb** your **anatomy** all over my **anatomy.**

Example: I really love the way you **run** your **tongue** all over my **tits.**

2. Asking for what you want:
Please **verb** my **anatomy** like you did last night.

Example: Please **lick** my **ass** like you did last night.

3. Hyperbolic Compliment:
That was the best **noun** I've ever had!

Example: That was the best **foot worship** I've ever had!

4. Guidance:
If you keep **verb** like that, I'm gonna **verb** so **adjective.**

Example: If you keep **pounding** me like that, I'm gonna **come** so **fast!**

5. Identity:
Yeah you like it when I **activity** you, don't you, you little **identity?**

Example: Yeah you like it when I **spank** you, don't you, you little **slut?**

6. Order:
I want you to come over and **verb** your **adjective, adjective noun** on my **anatomy.**

Example: I want you to come over and **sit** your **hot, dripping pussy** on my **face.**

7. Praise:
You look so **adjective** tonight, it makes me wanna **verb** you all over.

Example: You look so **delicious** tonight, it makes me wanna **bite** you all over.

8. Seduction:
I'm going to **verb** you and **verb** you until you **verb.**

I'm going to **lay** you out and **fist** you until you **cry.**

9. Domination and Submission:
Please may I have permission to **verb** your **noun, honorarium?**

Example: Please may I have permission to **lick** your **boots, Ma'am?**

10. Arousal:
It makes me **adjective** to watch you **verb.**

Example: It really makes me **hard** to watch you **dance.**

TABOO YOU

Usually, the very thing that makes dirty words so hot is the fact that they are taboo. Taboos can make forbidden acts extremely sexy, but they can also make us profoundly uncomfortable.

It's important to know the difference between adventuring outside of your comfort zone and getting into territories that make you unhappy. We learn our own boundaries by bravely exploring Remember that discomfort is subjective. There is no such thing as an intrinsically offensive word.

For example, my friend Monica is turned off by the word *cunt*. She associates the word with oppressive sexism and doesn't like to use it in bed to describe her vagina. On the other hand, the word *pussy* instantly turns her on. You could say it over and over again in bed and she would never tire of it.

Another friend of mine named Billy doesn't like to use the word *junk* to describe genitalia, because he doesn't want to equate bodies to garbage. My lover prefers to say *junk* regardless of the kind of genitalia she's referring to because she thinks of the term as gender-neutral and playful.

If you're trans, you may have very strong feelings about body vocabulary. For many gender-nonconforming folks, word choice is about more than arousal; it's also about identity affirmation. Many trans people experience feelings of dysphoria about their bodies. Using their chosen affirming language is a sign of respect as well as a sign that you want to turn them on. Cis folks also may have very strong, even triggering feelings around certain words. Regardless of gender identity, the way to be respectful is to know yourself and ask your partners about their preferences.

A trans male friend of mine named Josh likes to refer to the part of his anatomy he used to call his clitoris as his dick, and his favorite strap-on dildo as his

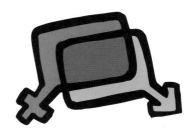

cock. He likes to be penetrated in either his "front hole" or his "back hole." Betty, a trans-female friend, tells me she loves for her strap-on to be called her "dick," while her own anatomy is affirmed as her "clit." Yet another guy I know likes when his asshole is being penetrated for it to be called his "pussy."

What are the words for your body that turn you on? What words are turnoffs? What do you want to hear in bed? What do you need to hear in bed? What do you need to *not* hear in bed? Know your answers to these questions so you can custom-make the dirty talk that works for you!

WHAT DO YOU DO IF YOUR PARTNER'S BUZZWORD IS YOUR BUZZKILL?

I have two good friends—let's call them Jules and George—who used to sleep together. Jules confessed that George would always say "I'm gonna nut!" right before orgasm. Jules couldn't describe what turned her off about it, but she found herself stifling laughter every time he said it. She didn't want to hurt his feelings, but she also didn't want to hear the verb *to nut* anymore.

My advice to her was this: Remember that George says "I'm gonna nut!" because it's his buzzword. Maybe in the past his partners have also been turned on by his enthusiasm. Or maybe nobody ever told him it was a phrase best kept to his private masturbation routine.

First, try to get used to new or unusual dirty talk, especially if this person is a casual sex partner. If you simply can't get over it, bring it up safely away from the act itself. You don't want George to become embarrassed whenever he has an orgasm, worrying that every woman he's been with has been secretly laughing at him. Put the emphasis on you: "I find the word *nut* distracting," or "I would find it so sexy if you said *come* instead of *nut*."

There's no reason to shame someone for his buzzword just because you find it silly.

Sometimes your partner's turn-on word is your turnoff. Just try to be kind about letting him or her know.

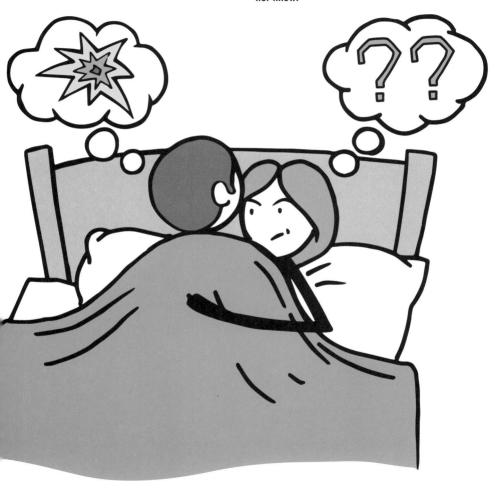

SWEET, SWEET FANTASY BABY

Sometimes the best way to get into dirty talk is to pretend to be someone else for a while. Playing a role is a chance to get into the "play" part of sex, to allow your inventiveness and theatricality to run wild. If costumes, props, or elaborate settings help you get into your scene, by all means, get creative.

If you want to check into a hotel to pretend to be a secretary meeting her boss for an illicit affair, or you want to rent a room in your local dungeon studio to live out your medieval torture scene, then do it! If a French maid outfit from your local boutique or an immersive rubber pig hood signals the beginning of playtime, go to town!

However, the most essential equipment here is your imagination. An entire scene or a detailed character backstory can emerge from the suggestion of simple dialogue. You don't need to break the bank or rely too much on gear to get all the benefits of living your fantasies. Simply suggest a character or role to your partner.

For example:

"Tonight I wanna be your dog!"

or

"You've been very bad, and as punishment I'm going to rub my pussy all over your face!"

A word about taboo: Often, pretending to be someone we're not requires us to play with complicated issues of right and wrong. For example, a real principal seducing his real student would be completely inappropriate, not to mention illegal. However, when two consenting adults *pretend* to be these roles, it's completely healthy. You don't become the character; rather, you enjoy what the character represents to you.

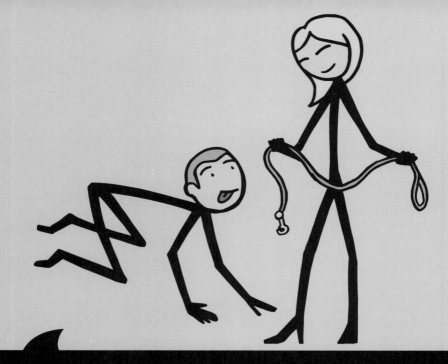

CUSTOMIZE THE FOLLOWING ROLE-PLAYS TO YOUR DESIRES
(the gender can always be switched for any of these)

Pool boy and desperate housewife

Eager puppy and expert trainer

Sultry super villain and captive superhero

Vicious vampire and mortal
star-crossed lover

Egotistical rock star and reckless groupie

College freshman being hazed for a
fraternity or sorority

Secretary blackmailing her boss

Complete strangers hooking up

Super-girlie slumber party

Professional athletes in the locker room

PERSONA AND IDENTITY

When is role-play more than role-play? When it becomes a sexual persona. Perhaps this is a character that gets you so hot that you like to play it again and again. Maybe it's a deeper expression of your personality or a dynamic that really helps your relationship. For example, you might be the domineering mistress in the bedroom, and your date may be a submissive boy. When you're in the grocery store, you're two egalitarian people shopping for produce, but in the bedroom you shift into your established personas. I know many people who have special names, protocols, or accessories such as collars that help them get into that special persona.

Another way to use identities as dirty talk is to use the power of demeaning words such as *slut, whore, bitch*, or *faggot*. For the exact same reason that taboo scenarios can be erotically charged, many people find it very sexy to be called something in the sheets that they wouldn't want to be called in the streets. The trick with making this consensual is very simple: the person who is being called a slut needs to be the one to ask for it.

PASSIONATE NONSENSE

Don't underestimate the power of nonsense. Dirty talk doesn't have to be expressed in any comprehensible human language. Those of us who live in apartments with thin walls, or have roommates or children, are used to keeping our voices down. If we grew up masturbating in secret in our rooms, we're used to stifling our own orgasmic cries.

If you want to get started verbalizing your passion and you really can't think of anything to say, try a vowel sound: *Aaa! Ooh! Uggh!*

You may be amazed by how giddy you feel when you growl, grunt, squeal, giggle, sigh, and moan.

Body language also counts as sexy communication. Make bold eye contact. Use a trick I've learned in many workshops: try looking deep into your partner's left eye with your left eye to create emotional empathy.

If you want to show your date that you're ready to get busy, spread your legs and run your hands along your thighs. Or bend over, arching your back and looking flirtatiously over your shoulder like a pin-up girl. Lean back, spreading your arms along the back of the couch. Anything that opens your body shows you are receptive to seduction.

TRUE ROMANCE CAN BE SEXY, TOO

Thank goodness we live in a world in which the idea of "meaningless" sex is totally outdated. Sex can *mean* so many different things. Sex can be two strangers who want to feel human connection for one night and never see one another again. Sex can be a hobby that two friends enjoy together because they're both really good at it!

Sex can be an expression of all different kinds of love, including marriage, partnership, friendship, or respect. For the right people, *I love you* can be the most arousing thing to say while you're coming. Or to be more specific, try one of the expressions of affection and intimacy at right:

I feel so safe with you.

You're the best boyfriend in the world.

You belong to me.

I need you.

I never want to be apart from you.

I want this moment to last forever.

Try incorporating your personal pet names into sex, or use one of these common ones:

Baby

Darling

Sweetheart

Honey

Angel

Babe

Sugar

Boo

Princess

Kitten

Finally, one of the most powerful words you can use in bed is right under your nose: your partner's name. When I hear my name in bed, I feel important to the person's experience. When I say someone's name while I'm coming, it's because I'm so obsessed with her, so incredulous that we're sharing something so mind-blowing, that I want to announce her name as if she has just won a prestigious award!

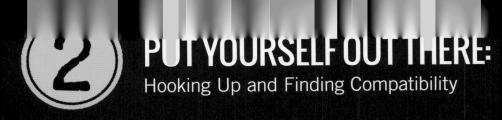

In today's world, many people use sites and apps such as OkCupid to meet dates, Grindr to hook up, 3ndr for threesomes, and Farmers Only for, well . . . farmers. The stereotype of the lonely loser who uses online dating because he can't connect in real life is a thing of the past.

This means that twenty-first-century dating is predicated on an annoying paradox. On one hand, you have a universe of possibility for hot sex and sweet love at your fingertips, right there in your personalized pocket computer. On the other hand, that infinite universe can be incredibly alienating, to the degree that you begin to think of each dating profile as a flat soulless character in a video game to which you are hopelessly addicted.

The trick to mastering this digital dating game involves taking advantage of all the opportunities without becoming overwhelmed or dehumanized. It may take a little self-discipline, but the tips and tricks in this chapter will help you learn proper etiquette and hopefully snag you some dates.

You'll need a few communication tools to navigate the world of online dating. You want to create a profile you're proud of, one that portrays you as the beautiful, charming superstar you know you are. You want to find profiles that will actually make good matches for you, whether it's for tonight or for a lifetime. You want to know just what to say to transform the hottie in that profile you're looking at now into tomorrow's perfect date.

You could find exactly what you're looking for. You could find something you didn't realize you were looking for. Your phone—the thing you use to call your mother and transfer funds from your savings to your checking account—can become a divining rod, leading you to your one true love or the lay of the century.

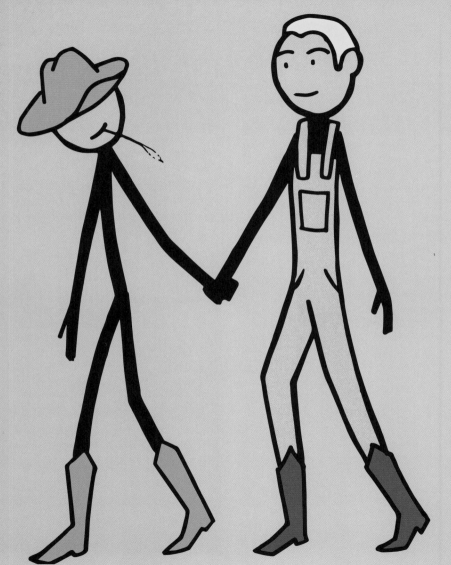

FIRST THINGS FIRST: LOVE YOURSELF

No, really.

Online dating provides so many options that you may be tempted to fill up your schedule with dates. Coffee dates before work. Cocktails immediately after work. Friday night movies, Saturday afternoon in the park, Sunday brunch. All the stimulation and excitement and potential to get lucky can seem too delicious to pass up.

If you masturbate (Seriously, hello people! Put this book down, go masturbate, and then we'll go from there; I promise you it will not make you go blind), then you already know that you don't need another human being to experience arousal. You can do that yourself, and it would be a privilege for someone else to participate in your pleasure!

For every weekend day you plan a date, plan a date for yourself. Exercise, read the paper, go shopping, cook a meal, work on an art project, or play a game. Be the kind of person you would want to date. You probably wouldn't want to go out with someone whose only hobby was dating.

Regardless of what you're looking for, you're more likely to find it when you project confidence in your own well-rounded life.

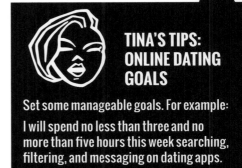

TINA'S TIPS: ONLINE DATING GOALS

Set some manageable goals. For example:

I will spend no less than three and no more than five hours this week searching, filtering, and messaging on dating apps.

I will work on trying to make at least one date happen this week.

I will go on no more than two dates this week.

CREATING YOUR PROFILE

At this point, most of us have some experience creating an online profile. You probably have a Facebook, LinkedIn, Twitter, or Google Plus account, and you probably have a MySpace and Friendster profile floating around locked with a password you can't remember. Representing yourself online to prospective employers or people who already love you is a snap compared to designing the perfect dating profile. What you say, and don't say, may vary from OkCupid to Tinder to other dating apps. The most important things to ask yourself are: What do I want, and what do I want to put out there?

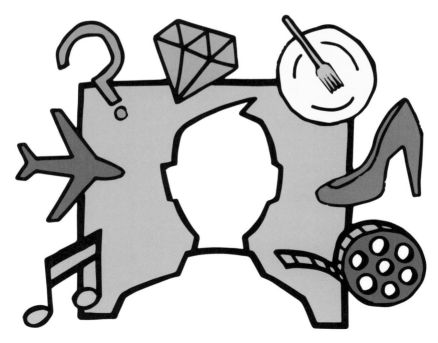

VISUALIZE YOUR PREY

Now that you're feelin' yourself, let's figure out what you're after. It's the twenty-first century, after all, and you have unprecedented freedom of choice! Get out your personal sexy journal from chapter 1: it's your time to dream. What happens in your fantasy world where you magically get everything you want?

Some things you may be on the hunt for:

A one night stand (or one morning sit, or one afternoon recline)

You're horny and you want hot sex delivered to your door like a motherfuckin' pizza! Maybe it's hotter when it's anonymous, and you don't even want to know his name. A little later in this chapter we'll talk about how to take care of yourself when you're enjoying the turn-on of getting naked with someone you barely know.

A dependable booty call

The booty call is a different species than the one-night stand. You and your booty call may get to know each other, or even become (gasp!) friends. Yet the focus of your relationship should always be hedonism, pleasure, and spontaneity. This is the person you meet up with for a beer and a slice before having wild monkey sex until the sun comes up. We'll also talk later on about how to be a great booty call.

Kink compatibility

Maybe you're a submissive seeking a Mistress to serve. Or you love to spank willing bottoms. Maybe you're into leather, electricity, or rope. You may want to try kink-specific sites such as FetLife, for these types of adventures.

Long-term commitment

There are an infinite number of relationship types, and it's important to know what you're looking for in a long-term partner. Nonmonogamy? Cohabitation? Joint bank accounts?

Monogamish-mash

Do you want to make sure everyone you date is open to a multiple-partner lifestyle? Are you in a couple, looking for a third party to play with? Are you that magical unicorn who wants to be the guest star in the bed of an existing couple? You don't have to list every fantasy you've ever had in your profile, but it's best to mention that you're open to ethically slutty situations.

Of course, you may be open to one or all of these options, or one that transforms into another. The trick is not to assume that other people's needs and boundaries are compatible with yours. It helps to be specific and intentional—none of that vague Prince Charming bullshit. This will make your matches easier to recognize.

Now think about what you value in a person. Don't be afraid to focus on the physical! It doesn't make you shallow to care about your partner's looks.

There is no such thing as conventionally attractive; everyone finds different things sexy. Do you love green eyes, sharp dressers, round bellies, or athletic legs?

As for personality, do you value kindness, good humor, chivalry, book smarts, street smarts, extroversion, or cultural tastes? Sometimes you can tell these things about a person from her profile, and sometimes you just have to take a chance and find out when you're face to face.

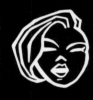

TINA'S TIPS: KEEP AN OPEN MIND

Now, the hardest part: be willing to throw all of these details out for the right person. We all know someone who is so set in his vision of the ideal girlfriend that he can't see a good thing when it's right under his nose. Keep an open mind about someone who may not seem like your "type."

WRITING YOUR OWN ADVERTISING COPY

Even once you've brainstormed and visualized the kind of relationship you want and the kind of person you want to have it with, writing your profile can seem like yet another daunting task. Simply choosing the pictures can be enough to make you want to get thee to a nunnery! Luckily, we have an entire chapter for the visual side, so let's focus on the words for now.

Take your time with your profiles (you may have slightly different profiles for different sites). Fill out the questions in a separate saved document on your computer so you can ruminate without the distraction of the app.

Imagine yourself as a character. This character is an accentuated, amplified version of you. Your character should have real flaws: show that you have dimension and can laugh at yourself. In a way, you're writing a little story. You want your text to be dynamic. Think about a character in a movie or TV show that always gets what she wants. Now fuse your personality with hers. Imagine yourself in her outfits and environments. How would she describe herself in a sultry voice-over?

How do you like to be perceived? For example, I love it when people compliment me on my tattoos, which I'm very proud of, or my blue eyes, which I feel show my personality. I always emphasize those traits in my profiles because it sends the message that it will make me feel good to be recognized in that way.

Sprinkle your profile with codes intended to gauge compatibility. For example, queers have developed an elaborate system of hanky codes that demonstrate what they're into, including whether they like to be on top or on bottom. Or it may be about a nonsexual interest like a favorite book, or a reference to your faith. Always remain open and remember that dating apps provide a chance to connect with people who may surprise you.

Ask your friends for profile critiques and instruct them to be brutally honest. Do the same for their profiles in return. It can be really challenging to know whether you're coming across as confident or arrogant, easygoing or a pushover, brilliant or pretentious. Be willing to make ongoing adjustments. Think of the relationship between your profile and the dates you have as a science experiment. If you're not having any luck for a few weeks, a simple tweak to your phrasing may attract exactly what you're after.

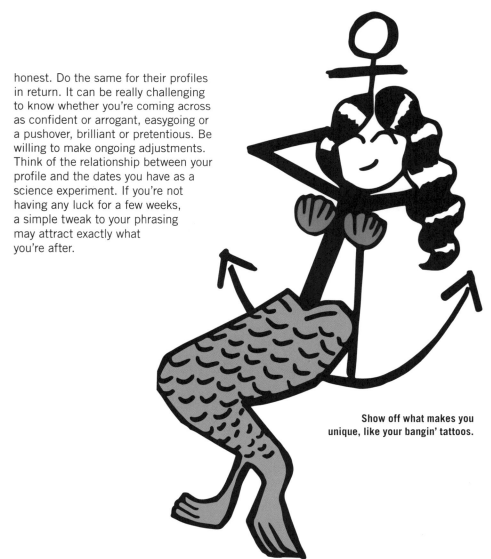

Show off what makes you unique, like your bangin' tattoos.

TINA'S GUIDE TO OPTIMIZING TIME ON APP CHATS

All right, your profile is composed, decorated, workshopped by your trusted council, and ready to get you laid! Now you have to learn to navigate *other* people's profiles, send out a few feelers, and manage the responses.

Step 1: Compose a Canned Response

Don't agonize over every syllable of every message. Say it out loud before you send it, so that it resembles the way you actually speak.

> Hiya gorgeous,
> Your profile is so great and I would love to get to know you better. Would you wanna grab a beverage sometime? If you're interested, hit me up! -Tina

Or:

> What's up? Your pictures and profile really stood out to me. I'd love to hang out when you've got some free time. Looking forward to it! -Tina

Step 2: Personalize

Now let's say I'm attracted to a girl's profile because she says she loves the outdoors and modern art. Personally, I like to skip the small chat and ask her out. I'll customize my canned response:

> Hiya gorgeous,
> Your profile is so great and I would love to get to know you better. I love Central Park too! Cherry Hill is my favorite spot. Would you wanna grab a lemonade with me there sometime? If you're interested, hit me up! -Tina

Or:

> What's up? Your pictures and profile really stood out to me. I've been meaning to go to the MOMA for a while, would you want to be my date? Looking forward to the idea! -Tina

Note how I acknowledge something from her profile, offering something genuine I have in common. Then I directly ask her for a date. It shows I'm observant, thoughtful, and ready to take the initiative.

Step 3: Keep It Up

A great interested response to my park invite could be:

Hi Tina!
It's so nice to hear from someone else who loves Sleater-Kinney as much as I do. Your idea for lemonade in the park sounds really dreamy, especially if I can bring a little whiskey to spike it with! Are you free Saturday afternoon? Send me a text-555.555.5555. 'Til then, Frankie

The crucial next step is to keep the conversation volleying.

What do I now know about this person?

- Her name is Frankie, and she has given me permission to call her that.

- She acknowledged something from my profile about our shared taste, which shows her mutual interest in me.

- She responded affirmatively to my suggestion for a date, and even threw her own twist on the idea!

- She gave me her digits! I'm going to contact her via text from now on.

Now, not all responses are going to make you fist pump in the air the way this one would. However, this should be the standard by which you gauge a response. Compared to this dream date, a response of simply "*Hey/Sure/Cool/Nice*" feels pretty rude, disrespectful, pointless, and inadequate, right?

In all exchanges over dating apps, always respond to something from the previous message and give the person something to respond to. If you're talking to someone and he leaves the conversation dead in the water, abandon that thread. Anyone worth dating will take the time to compose a thoughtful response.

If you *don't* hear back from someone after you've sent him the perfect cute message, do *not* follow up with another message. That's creepy. Let it go. Not everyone is going to be interested and/or available. Don't dwell on it. Disappointment is an important aspect of dating. The more you accept these little disappointments, the less they will feel like full-on rejection.

Step 4: Use Apps Exclusively to Establish Interest

Did you notice how Frankie's response in the above example offered her phone number and encouraged *me* to send a text from the get-go? I highly recommend that you get your conversation onto another mode of communication as soon as you can.

Do not engage in boring pointless small talk on OkC chat. Do not talk to people online just because you're lonely. Do not process serious emotions like rejection over messaging apps.

Don't be a creep. Even if you're only interested in sex, don't open with, *"wanna fuck?"* or *"u horny?"* and don't dignify such messages with a response either.

People tend to converse differently with different mediums. I don't talk logistics over Twitter DMs and I don't break up over Facebook chat. When I start texting on my private text messages with someone I met on a dating app, the structural cues remind me I'm talking to a person, not just playing a horny video game.

TINA'S TIPS: DON'T WASTE YOUR OWN TIME ON SELF-DEFEATING INTERNAL MONOLOGUES

There is no such thing as "out of my league," or "he'll never write me back so what's the point?" in online dating. If you like the looks of someone's profile, just go for it! Putting yourself out there teaches you the discernment you need to optimize your search, and being disappointed helps build emotional muscles. What do you really have to lose? Absolutely nothing.

TINA'S COMMANDMENTS
FOR ONLINE DATING COMMUNICATION

1. Thou shalt be self-disciplined with thy online cruising.

Sometimes opening your favorite dating apps can be as tempting as scrolling through your Instagram feed. Except instead of looking at your friend's adorable puppies playing in the snow, you're sifting through the profiles of actual people looking to meet actual other people. The excitement of possibility and the dopamine rush of being contacted by someone cute can be downright addicting. Before you know it, you're spending more time swiping left or right on Tinder than you are cultivating human connection.

Set yourself a time limit for the day and stick to it. Say, opening no more than three times per day or no more than an hour total. You're not likely to find more of what you're looking for by spending more time on the apps.

Cruise better, not longer.

2. Thou shalt be assertive.

Hands down, the most effective way to get what you want is to develop a clear, assertive, fun online persona who reads people's social cues and respects their boundaries.

If OkCupid is a party, then this ideal persona is the one who smiles, makes eye contact, sticks out her hand, and says, "Hi! I'm Tina!" If that person doesn't respond to her, she has plenty of confidence to go talk to someone else. Make the first move. Don't be manipulative or coy.

3. Thou shalt be unwavering in thy boundaries.

A boundary isn't a boundary if you're always rescinding it. Set your own rules for intimacy and stick to them. You may say no sex on the first date, or no sex if the first date involves alcohol. Or you may go directly for the sex, but hold a firm line about sleepovers until the third date. Maybe you have red flags regarding lifestyle choices, like you won't seriously date someone who is separated but not divorced, doesn't have a job, or smokes cigarettes.

Let your date know about these boundaries ahead of time, and be consistent with them. If someone triggers your red flags, even if it's just a feeling in your gut, go with it and let her down politely but firmly.

4. Thou shalt not use dating app chats for sexual stimulation.

Don't masturbate while chatting with potential dates, and don't try to engage people to sext with you before meeting up. There is always a chance you'll find someone who only wants to have cybersex, but it's far more likely you'll end up being an insincere creep. Don't continue to send sexually suggestive messages to someone who has not responded. At best, this is false pretense—at worst, abuse.

A charming sex worker—who will negotiate time and limits to provide you with erotic entertainment—is always just a mouse click away. Do not attempt to get your kicks from people who are searching in earnest for noncommercial human connection online.

5. Thou shalt not obsessively check thy messages while waiting for a response.

We've all done it. Do yourself a favor and try to wean yourself off the habit. You're causing yourself a whole lot of unnecessary grief. What's worse is that it keeps you from being able to spot good things when they actually come to you.

6. Thou shalt not feel guilty about not writing everyone back.

I had a friend who quit OkCupid after a month; she said it was too time-consuming to write everyone back. She was a sweet, intelligent, gorgeous woman living in Brooklyn, getting hundreds of messages a week. She felt like she was being rude and letting them all down if she didn't respond, even if it was to say she wasn't interested.

You *are not* obligated to respond to everyone who reaches out to you, no more than a company needs to feel bad about not responding to everyone who applies for a position. If someone doesn't impress you with his first message, he should spend his time honing his flirting skills to find someone he's compatible with. It's not your job to train him. Everyone on online dating should understand that no response means a polite "Thanks, but no thanks." This shouldn't dissuade you from continuing to put yourself out there!

Besides, rejecting people with compassion and being rejected is a powerful way to learn healthy relationship habits. When we get used to micro-rejections we realize it's not the end of the world when someone decides he or she doesn't want to date us.

7. Thou shalt not waste thy time on correcting the etiquette of people thou hast no interest in dating.

You might as well accept that the minute you sign onto these sites you are going to be assaulted by creeps, misogynists, and trolls. Believe me, you are going to want to give these assholes a piece of your mind.

They will not hear you. If you really must correct someone's etiquette, do it quickly and then disengage. You have better things to do, like finding people to date who aren't douche bags.

8. Thou shalt be transparent about thine intentions.

Don't pretend you're looking for a monogamous commitment when you're exclusively interested in no-strings-attached sex. Don't lead someone on with the promise of sex because that's the only way you think you can get her to date you. People looking for hookups should find other compatible matches who are looking for hookups. Daters should meet daters. Be up front, and I promise you'll find more of what you're looking for.

My friend Suzanne has a great tip: Don't message someone after midnight unless it's for a hookup.

9. Thou shalt not be afraid of the block button; it is thy friend.

It bears repeating: some people are assholes, and nothing you can do will change that. When people reveal themselves to be racist, sexist, homophobic, transphobic, or simply rude, just block them and move on. You're too good to stoop to the level of bullies and bigots.

10. Thou shalt be kind.

Then there are the perfectly nice people you interact with online who are just not compatible with you. Treat them with dignity. It may seem like there are no consequences to online cruelty, but the world is just better when everyone practices the Golden Rule: treat others as you would like to be treated.

This means being firm with people you're not interested in, and open with the people you want to get to know. At any rate, it's a well-known fact that those who exhibit common human decency give the best head.

THE FIRST DATE

All the digital gauging in the world is no substitute for chemistry. You may click, as they say, on the first date. And you may not. You may be interested, and the other person may not be, or the other way around. He may have communicated well online but in person he's a dud. Don't be hard on yourself if the date feels like a waste of time. Every mismatch teaches you what to look for and what to avoid in your future hunts.

If it doesn't work out, remember to be kind. This person may not be right for you but he's definitely right for someone else. The same goes for agreeing to more dates when you know you're not interested: you actually are not doing him any favors by stringing him along.

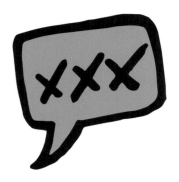

A LITTLE LIGHT STALKING NEVER HURT ANYBODY...

Is it still a blind date when you know exactly what the person looks like?

Blind dates, of course, are a quaint idea from an era long before our age of socially acceptable Google stalking. Doing a little background check on your date isn't a bad idea at all. You can find out more about her that you can use to warm up the conversation, or you may learn something that will prevent you from even having a first date.

It's best to be subtle about all this. Don't specifically mention the stalking. Just because we all do it doesn't mean we want to hear about it.

Just be fair, and keep in mind that the way people present themselves online may be more stiffly professional (a.k.a. *boring*) than they are socially. Or that the way they make inside jokes with their friends on social media isn't necessarily how they would conduct themselves in a romantic relationship. Your date contains multitudes, just like you do!

TINA'S TIPS: AVOID BACKHANDED COMPLIMENTS

When meeting up with someone you met online, always say, "You look great tonight," instead of, "You are so much better looking in person than in your photo!" If someone tells me the latter, all I hear is that I'm not photogenic and that I'm bad at picking good profile pictures.

ALWAYS MEET IN PUBLIC

Anyone who wants to do otherwise isn't trustworthy. Even if all you want to do is hook up, anyone worth hooking up with will understand why you would want to be seen together in public before you're alone behind closed doors. This also gives you a chance to see whether you have the same spark in person that you did over digital exchange.

Even if it's spontaneous and late at night, always meet in a bar for a drink or grab coffee at a diner. Have a polite list of reasons you may need to leave after an hour or one drink. Have a friend agree to call you at a certain time to give you an opening.

BE A GOOD LISTENER

You know when you go on a date and the person places his phone on the table like a beeping, glowing security blanket? Do not do this. It's distracting and insulting.

Be present when you're on a date. Don't keep your dating apps open trying to figure out the next thing you're doing.

Also, skip the small talk! You've already read each other's profiles. Your first date is a chance to get each other talking about subjects you both genuinely enjoy.

When I'm going out with someone new, I occasionally find myself wondering, "Is he on this date just so he can talk about himself, or does he actually want to get to know me?"

Plan ahead for your nervousness or excitement by asking your date something specific about her. If her profile interested you at all, it must have given you an extensive guide to her interests, history, and identity. This is your chance to see whether she measures up in person. When she asks about you, take your turn. Don't be afraid to get real!

SOME GREAT LINES TO TRANSITION THE DATE TO SOMEWHERE MORE PRIVATE

"Wanna come over and make out?"

"I'd love to spend the night with you."

"OMG, you've never seen *Jurassic Park*? Come to my place and we can watch it on my laptop!" (I used this one constantly in college!)

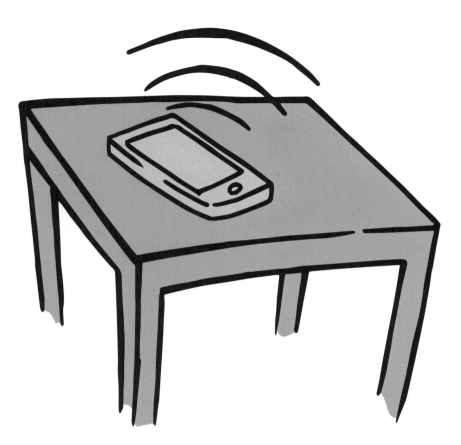

There is nothing ruder than a date whose eyes keep drifting to his or her buzzing phone. Put your phone on silent and put it away.

HOW TO DISCUSS SAFE SEX

Listen. I know how excruciating it can be to have a discussion about safe sex before you go to bed with somebody. I know because I'm a proud slut, and I've had those conversations literally hundreds of times. At times it has been like pulling teeth to get the right words out, but the sex is always so much better when I do.

If you practice your lines, and know your status and needs, then we're talking about five minutes of potential awkwardness that opens you up for an entire night of uninhibited passion. Fair trade, if you ask me. Personally, the only people I want to allow the privilege of getting naked and filthy with me are the people who are grown-up and responsible enough to be excited by these conversations.

TRY SOME OF THESE TIPS TO MAKE THIS PART SEXIER:

"I would really love to invite you over tonight. Let's get a few things out of the way first so we can relax."

"Do you know what really turns me on? Safe sex. Seriously. Because it's safe, and because it's sex!"

Use body language. Touch your date's hand, arm, or thigh. Scooch closer on the bar bench so the sides of your butts are touching. Make eye contact, even if you have to break it to smile and look down in shyness or sigh and look up coyly from time to time.

WHAT TO TALK ABOUT
BEFORE YOU GET NASTY TOGETHER

BIRTH CONTROL

If there's any chance that one of your anatomies can knock the other's up, you need to let each other know where you stand. Is there hormonal birth control or an IUD in the mix? Would you like to use a barrier for intercourse regardless?

WHAT YOU'RE LOOKING FOR RIGHT NOW

Fuck buddy? Love? Marriage? Baby carriage? These things always change, but you'll save yourself a ton of grief by getting on the same page about what you both want in the immediate future.

STIS AND TESTING

Ideally, anyone who is sexually active will be able to proclaim her chlamydia, syphilis, gonorrhea, and HIV status as of the past fourteen days. Contact your local clinic to find out the most affordable way to keep your status up to date.

BARRIER PROTECTION PREFERENCES

Whether to use condoms, gloves, female condoms, lube, or dental dams is a decision you should make well before you go on a date. Know whether you require a barrier for oral, vaginal, and anal sex, whether you have a latex allergy and require a nonlatex condom/glove, and whether someone's STI status influences your decision to use a barrier. Make safer sex sexier by drizzling lube, snapping a glove as you pull it over your wrist, or putting a condom on with your lips and tongue!

MONOGAMY STATUS

Are you in a primary relationship that's open? Are you looking for a monogamous commitment? Do you have multiple partners and want to keep it that way? If any of these variations or more is true, you have a responsibility to disclose and a right to know!

THE SILENT ALARM

Sometimes there's nothing hotter than anonymous sex. Apps allow you to custom order hookups just like you can choose your grocery delivery. The catch is that you may decide to invite someone to your house, or head to his, when you're thinking with the organs between your legs instead of the one between your ears.

I absolutely endorse the excitement of consensual objectification, and I don't want anyone to live in fear of the one bad apple in an orchard of ripe delicious fruits. One of my tried-and-true techniques to help mitigate hookup risks (in addition to several others listed elsewhere in this chapter) is the Silent Alarm.

It bears repeating that you must always meet your date at a diner or hotel lobby before going somewhere private. Make sure at least one trusted friend knows the address where you're meeting up and where the hookup is going down.

Always tell your date that you need to make a call right when you arrive and that your friend is expecting to hear from you again later that night or in the morning. This sends a clear message that someone knows where you are and cares about your fate.

Here's how the Silent Alarm works: You and a friend agree on a code. For example, my Silent Alarm buddy and I have the following code:

- "Let's get brunch tomorrow" = everything's actually fine
- "Let's get drinks this week" = call the cops
- "Everything's fine" = call the cops
- No call from me = call the cops

This accommodates for the worst-case scenario in which the date turns out to have less than honorable intentions, forcing you under duress to call your friend to say you're fine.

I have been very lucky in that I have never had to say anything other than, "Let's get brunch," with a big horny grin when I call my friend. However, I have had friends who have needed to "activate" their Silent Alarm, or who have had dates who have suspiciously backed out when they find out someone is waiting for my friend's call. The Silent Alarm helps you experience the turn-on of hookups while reducing stranger danger.

THE FOLLOW-UP

There are those who worry that online dating is creating a culture of "easy-cum-easy-go" attitudes toward dating. In my mind, our digital tools give us the chance to communicate more efficiently in unique scenarios of modern love and sex.

My friend Mariana recently told me about a great experience she had with a guy. They met on OkCupid, had a fun date, and went home together for what she describes as truly exceptional sex. They hooked up a few times after that, and she was pretty sure she wanted to keep the relationship primarily sexual. Then one day she received a text from him:

> Hey Mariana. You're amazing and I have had so much fun with you lately! I've started dating someone else seriously, so I can't hook up with you anymore. But I would still love to hang out as friends if you're down. Give me a call anytime. -Toby

Let's break this down: Apparently, Toby was seeing several women casually, and then started to get serious and monogamous with one of them. He could have just stopped calling all his other dates. Instead, he did something considerate to his new girlfriend *and* all the rest of the women he was seeing.

By sending a flattering, clear message, he gave Mariana the gift of not wondering why he wasn't returning her booty calls. He saved her from the agony of playing the guessing game: *Was it something I said? Was the sex really as good as I thought it was?* This may have soured her on the memory of what was otherwise some mutually beneficial fun times.

An added bonus for Toby: If he and his girlfriend ever break up and Mariana is still available, she will be much more inclined to sleep with him again because of his considerate message.

I GET BY WITH A LITTLE HELP FROM . . .

Friends . . . remember them? The people you didn't need a fancy app to find? Of course your friends absolutely want you to be happy, to find love and orgasms and whatever else you're after.

We all know the stereotype of the fair-weather friend who stops hanging out with her crew as soon as she gets into a relationship . . . and then comes crawling back needing care and attention after every breakup. Maybe you've had a few friends like that, and maybe you've *been* a friend like that once or twice. It might help to be able to spot whether *you're dating* someone like that.

The problem with this pattern is that the fair-weather friend doesn't look for balance. She becomes addicted to the merry-go-round ride of dates, thinking that her needs will be met that way.

This is why it's so important to understand what you truly value. If you've had a lot of hookups lately but still feel unsatisfied, it's not because casual sex is inherently meaningless. It may be that what you were really after was adventure, or physical touch, or somebody to talk to honestly. You can get that from your friends. Doing so could refresh your spirit, keeping you open and ready to find the romance and sexual connection you're after from your dates.

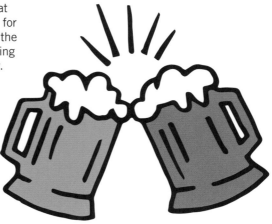

TINA'S GUIDE TO BEING A GOOD BOOTY CALL

1. **Be clear that's what you're after and what you're offering.** Make your intentions sexy and appealing. They don't have to sound clinical or like a business transaction.

> Hey gorgeous, I'm busy with work the rest of the week but I could be all yours tonight if you're free.

2. **Try to find something you have in common to talk about besides sex:** sports, movies, books, politics, science, food, fashion, whatever!

3. **Ideally, get tested every fourteen days and have your test results at the ready.** Be clear and on the same page about birth control and barriers.

> I want you to know I do have herpes (like one in six Americans!), but I haven't had an outbreak in two years.

> Just so you know I have a latex allergy so I'll be bringing my own condoms! ;)

4. **See each other no more than once a week.** If you see each other more than that, be ready to accept that you might be more than booty calls.

> Thanks for the invite for tonight but I'm still sore from seeing you last weekend. Are you free next Sunday tho?

5. **Extend common human decency.** Bring each other a freaking glass of water. Introduce your booty call to your roommates.

6. **If you're dealing with your own internalized shame about being slutty, don't project it onto your booty call.** Nobody likes a hypocrite.

7. **Don't be a flake.** Be on time. Return text messages, even if it's to say,

> Sorry, babe, I'm in for the night, but I can't wait to sit on your face this weekend.

8. **Good fences make good neighbors.** Have good boundaries. Don't invite your booty call to be your date to your best friend's wedding or to go on a weeklong road trip to your dad's house for Thanksgiving. Again, if you do want to do these things, be ready to accept that you might be more than booty calls.

9. **Spend the night if you both enjoy that, and offer each other food and coffee in the morning, but don't let sleepovers become epic brunches become afternoon sex become sleepovers** . . . *If you do want to do these things*, be ready to accept (you guessed it!) that you might be more than booty calls.

10. **Be good in bed.** Just because someone is a fuck buddy who is only a text message away doesn't mean she is just a living breathing sex toy. Care about your booty call's orgasms. Be adventurous together!

11. **If you start dating someone else seriously or you lose interest in that person and you're not available anymore, just let him know in a kind and encouraging way.** It is way better to get that message than to think someone is still on your roster and is rejecting you. He shared his genitals with you, so give him the dignity of freeing up his time to pursue someone who wants him back.

12. **Do not ignore someone for months and then text her for sex.**

13. **If you have a dozen people you call when you're feeling randy, go you!** But please keep them straight. I roll my eyes so hard when I've told someone I'm out of town and I keep getting the same canned come-on group text from him.

14. **Accept that objectification can be awesome when it's consensual.**

You are just a piece of meat I want to tenderize.

15. **Expect all of this behavior of your booty call in return. Delete his number if he doesn't live up to your expectations.**

EVERY DATE IS A DIGITAL AUDITION

The technology for meeting people may have changed, but the possibilities for both love and heartbreak never will. Some people get real lucky, but most people are gonna kiss a lot of frogs before they meet a prince. Think of every "frog" as a chance to learn what works for you and what doesn't.

Consider the dating game like ongoing film role auditions. Your goal is to be a movie star. You're a hard worker and you've been studying method-acting techniques. You have to keep auditioning over and over and over again, and you are going to get used to rejection.

Sometimes the person who was cast instead of you baffles you completely. Sometimes you know that you would definitely have been better for the part (and all your besties assure you this is correct).

Yet every time you audition, you have to take a deep breath, lift your head up high, and read your lines like the shining superstar you know you are. It may seem like you keep trying and trying, and that you deserve to just find the job you're after already. But there are no guarantees in life. As soon as you accept that you're not entitled to love or sex, you start to feel free.

Sooner or later, you're going to land the role of a lifetime. You're going to stare into the eyes of your costar and hear some far-off voice yell your cue:

"Action!"

TINA'S TIPS:
HASH IT OUT

If you don't already, please start talking with your friends about sex. Throw out any stale ideas you may have about what is polite conversation. Good friends listen with curiosity and don't judge. We need to bounce our fantasies and neuroses off of the people we love, respect, and trust. All the dating etiquette books in the world can't compare to the bespoke advice you'll get from your friends who know when you need classic soothing comfort and when you need customized tough love.

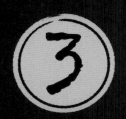

DISCOVER THE JOYS OF SEXT:
Using Technology to Stay Turned On

Dear readers, I need to make a confession. I'm not really all that digitally savvy. I've read far too much dystopian science fiction to trust any technology outright. This usually results in me carrying around, say, the last cassette tape Walkman in existence long after it's gone out of style. But when I cave and begin using a modern-day gadget, I realize how lucky I am to have it and try to use it for good, not evil. And I always start by figuring out how to bend it to my raunchy needs.

Give me your phone number and I'll send you a hardcore text. Mark your chatting status to "Available" and I'll make sure you have to hide your boner under your desk at work. I'm naturally foul-mouthed and I tend to have conversations with people who are similarly lewd.

You may not be quite as much of a total perv as me, but you can still learn how to use technology to turn yourself and your partners on!

A note on instructions and terminology: I imagine most of this will be transferable regardless of your device. Even if you don't have a smartphone, you can probably do most of the sexting and picture sending we're going to go over in the next few chapters. If your phone is ancient and slow, you know what they say about antici . . . pation.

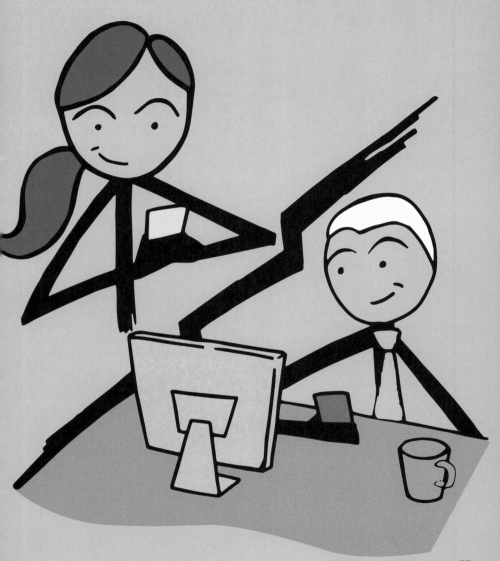

SEXTUAL HEALING

What is a sext? My definition of sexting encompasses any sexually themed message sent on an SMS service, instant-messaging chat, or email, especially when the purpose of that message is to erotically stimulate yourself and the recipient.

There are two main kinds of sexting:

1. Messages that are meant to be seductive, suggestive, or flirtatious

2. Messages that are meant to be read while masturbating

We're going to go over all the ways to send the best version of both kinds.

If you've had a bad experience with sexting, don't give up on the whole possibility. If everyone who ever had lousy sex swore off the act forever, we would be a nation of celibates.

CONVERSATIONAL BABY STEPS

You'll be able to apply the IRL techniques you learned in chapter 1 to your dirty digital dispatches. In fact, you may feel more comfortable typing out your wicked thoughts and sending them through your device. Maybe you're not ready to say, *"Your pussy is so perfect,"* or *"You're making my nipples hard,"* out loud, but you can certainly work up the nerve to send it in a text.

Compose and perfect your explicit sentences from a comfortable private space behind a screen. Once you've sent the text, and gotten positive feedback, you may start to feel bolder about saying it in person!

MAKING THE FIRST MOVE

So how do you know the moment is right to send a sexy message?

Use the same judgment you would with your partner when you're both in the same room. Most people prefer that their date does not shove his fingers in without so much as a kiss or a "How was your day, babe?" The same goes for sexting. Hint at your horniness. Get a feel for your partner's mood.

It's worth mentioning that sometimes we *do* want to be shoved against a wall or to rip someone's clothes off in the heat of passion. The sext equivalent of that might be a complete out-of-the-blue message asking, *"Do you miss my hard cock?"* or *"Are you still swollen from last night?"*

The thrill, the instant exhilaration of going from neutral to fifth gear, is a wonderful erotic technique that simply must be reserved for relationships with people you know well. If you're wondering how you know when to put out those inner bad-boy dominant moves, simply ask yourself, "Do I really believe this person will be turned on by this?"

Otherwise, it never hurts to build things slowly and deliberately.

GREAT OPENING SEXTS

- I've been very bad today.
- I can't stop thinking about you.
- I'm wearing that dress you like.
- I want you to be rough with me tonight.
- I'm craving your touch.

TINA'S TIPS:

DEVISE A CODE

It can be challenging to read your partner's mood when you only have her words on a screen to go by. One technique to signal that you're amenable to digital sexy times is to establish code sentences, pet names, and safe words.

For example, let's say I want to sext with my boyfriend while he's at work. I might send him a text calling him *Mi Amor*, a name I only use when I'm feeling randy. If he replies calling me *Mon Cheri*, then I know it's on!

We could also have coded sentences, such as *Hot out today, isn't it?* If he replies, *Actually, it's really cold at the office right now*, then I know he is too distracted to sneak off into the bathroom to take a picture of his dick for me.

Come up with the codes or safe words that are right for you and your partner: Red (Stop), Yellow (Slow), and Green (Go!) are always dependable choices.

USE DIFFERENT
RULES FOR DIFFERENT TECHNOLOGIES

One of the best ways to make your sexting effective is to determine different communication styles for different technology. Misunderstandings and crossed emotional wires occur most often when we think we've expressed A, but it's been interpreted as B. The alienation of technology only exacerbates this.

Here are my rules:

- I don't have serious conversations over G-chat (especially if my partner is at work).

- I avoid logistical conversations over hookup apps. Instead, switching to text shows I'm ready to meet up, moving away from the cruising zone.

- I find out whether my text buddy locks his phone or has push notifications turned off. If not, then I do not send unsolicited explicit texts that his roommate could read.

- While traveling or when in a long-distance relationship, I make time for FaceTime, not just text or phone calls, so I can see my partner's O face.

- I engage in nothing more than friendly banter or flirting over Facebook, Twitter, or other more general social networks.

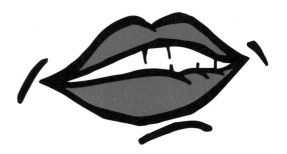

BE A TIME TRAVELER

We are all able to compartmentalize our conversations these days. I've sexted while riding a bus, standing on a sidewalk, and sitting in a meeting. I've even paid exorbitant Wi-Fi fees to sext on a plane.

So it's important to remember that although you may be snuggled up on your couch sipping a glass of Malbec, completely transfixed by your favorite sext conversation, your boo may be in that meeting, catching that train, or crossing the street. You don't want her to be hit by a car mid-text, no matter how hot the conversation! You definitely don't want her to lose her job because she didn't know when to divert her attention. Be patient if she doesn't get back to you for a few minutes. If you're feeling neglected mid-turn-on, get yourself off and text:

> You got me so hot I had to rub one out. I'll be waiting for you when you get back to your phone.

If you're the one multitasking, try not to leave someone hanging. Let your boo know what you're up to. Offer a

disclaimer early in the conversation that explains any anticipated radio silence. Try simply:

> Hey btw, I may have to disappear for a second to switch my laundry out. Don't you dare stop touching yourself! I'll brb.

Don't read too much into the "awareness indicator" if your phone has one (a.k.a. the shimmering ellipses bubble or italicized "Tina is typing . . ." line). It's there to create a sense of pacing in your written conversation that approximates verbal conversation. More often than not, it just produces anxiety and a sense of an awkward silence. Condition yourself not to read too much into those menacing *dot dot dots* because it will only cause you agony.

Finally, be aware that different people have different inclinations toward digital multitasking. If neither you nor your partner can sext on the run, make time to send each other hot messages when you're both relaxing at the end of a long day.

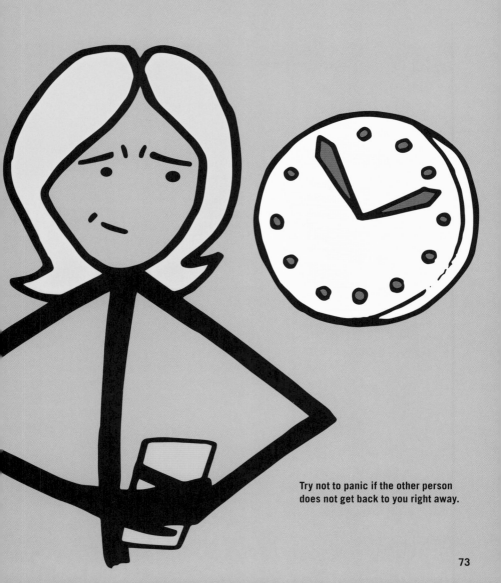

Try not to panic if the other person does not get back to you right away.

FOR HEAVEN'S SAKE, CHANGE YOUR SETTINGS TO NO PREVIEW

In chapter 4, we're going to have a good long exploration of the subject of privacy. When it comes to explicit texts, the rule is simple—set your lock screen so that it doesn't preview your text messages.

On an iPhone, go to Settings > Notification Center > Messages. Toggle Show Preview to OFF.

This will save you the inappropriate experience of your boss seeing that you're sexting, *I need to choke on your cum*, or the embarrassment of your mom grabbing your phone to search for directions and seeing a message from your girlfriend saying, *As soon as you walk in the door I want you on the floor so I can sit on your face.*

YOUR PHONE IS LIKE YOUR BEDROOM

Privacy is important in an oversharing world. I'm always horrified when I see people using each other's phones to check movie times or to look up the definition of a word.

To be honest, I think this because the background of my phone is usually the naked butt of someone special, and the owner of that butt is more often than not texting me something about what she wants to do to *my* butt.

It's a privilege to have a personal computer in your pocket, and we shouldn't take it for granted. However, I advise you to think of your phone as a space to which you have the right to shut the door.

Of course, it's a sign of trust to give someone the key to your apartment or the password to your phone. It's also a sign of trust to *not* give it—if you're comfortable not having your date's password, then it means you feel secure that she has nothing to hide.

IS SEXTING CHEATING?

Precisely what constitutes "cheating" varies from person to person and couple to couple. I think of cheating as anything deceptive that goes outside the negotiated rules of a relationship. If I have an agreement of sexual nonmonogamy with my partner, then I'm free to sext away—but it would be inconsiderate to do so while I'm on the couch watching TV next to her.

A good rule of thumb when making any fidelity decision is to put the shoe on the other foot. If you're considering sending an explicit text to your ex, ask yourself how you would feel if you found out your partner had done the same. If the idea makes you feel betrayed, then it's probably inconsiderate of you to do it.

Regardless of your arrangement, it would be a mistake to think of text exchanges as somehow "less real" or "not as serious" as face-to-face interactions. As we learn from constant political and celebrity scandals, philandering online can bring you just as much humiliation as actually having sex with someone who isn't your partner, and it can also be just as painful to the ones you love.

VOICE RECOGNITION TEXT

"I'm so out of shoes." Thanks, Siri.

I don't recommend using Siri or other voice recognition software to sext, because so much can be lost in translation. You just end up sending messages like, *I want to linger am now* or, *I'm so out of shoes*, more confusing than arousing.

WHOM SHOULD YOU SEXT?

The Internet can certainly facilitate wonderfully low-stakes erotic interactions, such as exchanging dick pics with strangers on Craigslist. However, it's important to distinguish between fantasy and reality by asking yourself the following question: How will this online interaction have concrete consequences in my life and the lives of others?

I have a friend named Amy who had an affair for several months with a coworker at her office job. Here's the catch: the affair was conducted entirely over G-chat and text message. In fact, the two of them barely interacted face to face, which certainly heightened the clandestine thrill of their raunchy exchanges. Amy explained to me that ordinarily she would know better than to indulge in a steamy office romance; she simply thought it "didn't count" because they weren't having real-life sex. When the relationship fizzled

out, they experienced the full force of awkwardness when they had to continue to interact as coworkers. Amy bemoaned, "I'm getting all the grief, and I didn't actually even get laid!"

The Internet doesn't magically transform a dumb situation into appropriate behavior. If you wouldn't engage in an unethical or inadvisable relationship in the physical world, don't use the digital mediation as an excuse. This goes for sexting someone underage, sexting someone in a monogamous relationship, sexting while operating heavy machinery, and sexting compulsively to the detriment of the rest of your life.

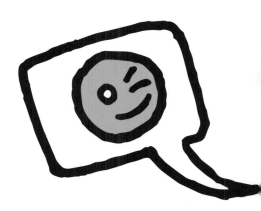

DOUBLE-CHECK THAT YOU'RE SEXTING THE RIGHT PERSON

Lord knows that half the fun of sexting is getting carried away and losing control. But if you are in any way toggling among tasks, take a breath and double-check before you click Send. This is another of the many reasons one should not sext while walking down the street or driving a car.

DON'T USE SOMEONE FOR SEXT

Do not sext with someone who wants to date you, but with whom you have no intention of actually meeting up in real life.

This is called leading someone on, and it's not cute.

SEXTING: WHAT IS IT GOOD FOR?

Sexting is a versatile activity and a useful tool for many types of relationships. Make the most of every sext session.

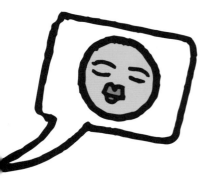

MASTURBATE TO YOUR TEXT CONVERSATIONS

I love to take screenshots of explicit conversations I've had and use them to work myself up. I definitely use sexy pictures for this, too, and we'll discuss that more in chapter 4. Sometimes I receive horny messages when I'm not in a position to touch myself; nevertheless, I enjoy the turn-on of feeling flustered and getting off harder later.

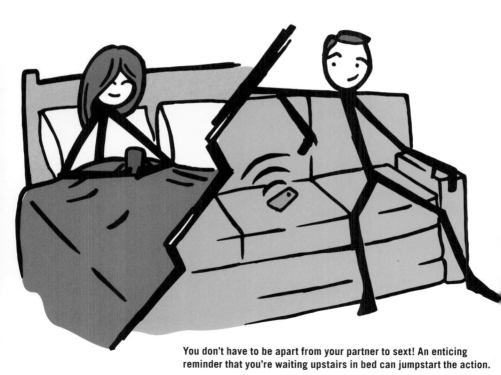

You don't have to be apart from your partner to sext! An enticing reminder that you're waiting upstairs in bed can jumpstart the action.

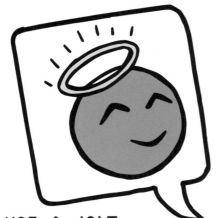

USE A JOLT OF INDECENCY TO BRIGHTEN UP A BORING SITUATION

It would seem that it is increasingly socially acceptable to thumb around on your phone in most environments. While I personally encourage everyone to be present and unplugged at restaurants, on commutes, or in school, a strategically sent sexy text can brighten up otherwise tedious undertakings.

For example, take your phone to the restroom during dinner with family or a long lecture. Steal this moment of seclusion to scroll through some racy messages and send some back. It may just inject your mind with so much new energy to help you make it through the rest of your day.

Want to be nice? Or naughty? A persona can make for a hot sexting session.

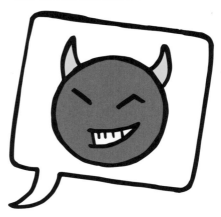

USE THAT CONTRAST BETWEEN NAUGHTY AND ORDINARY TO YOUR ADVANTAGE

Sometimes the sexiest thing about a sext is the fact that you're reading something rude while you're in otherwise polite company. If you take precautions explained in this chapter (code words, locked screens, remaining present), then you should feel free to make one another squirm with secret thrills.

HOW TO SEXT BETTER

Sexting requires more than a few *hey babys* and dick pics. Sexting is a skill! Hone your dirty mind with these useful tips.

Choose Your Own Adventure Erotica: There is no shortage of exciting porn in the world, and something on the market for anyone's tastes. (Side note: Please pay for the porn you enjoy, especially if you want to support the production of feminist, ethical, and independent productions.)

Adult entertainment can relieve stress and just plain make us happy. Yet nothing beats a customized stream of erotic stimulation created live for your pleasure!

Bridge the Distance: Have you ever dated someone who lived in a different city, state, or country? Do you frequently travel for work? Maybe you and your partner simply live on opposite sides of town. If so, sexting can be an amazing way to make your long-distance relationship feel erotically close.

Even if you're not in the same room for days, weeks, or even years, you can continue to stimulate each other's imaginations from afar.

Turn Yourself On! Too often we imagine that, especially for women, sending a sext is a chore or a service we do for someone else. In fact, saying dirty words can be just as arousing as hearing them, and typing dirty messages can be just as arousing as receiving them.

Imagine sexting as the digital equivalent of a striptease. Once you send that suggestive message, you have your boo wrapped completely around your finger. Think of the power this gives you!

Tease from Afar: Imagine your boo is at work. You send him a message saying you're masturbating right now. Now all he can think about is your naked body.

Here's a story from a friend of mine that encapsulates how hot it can be to distract your partner with a sext:

"I know my boyfriend likes to be teased and tormented a bit, and I like to do that with text messages when we're apart. Once he told me he had to masturbate immediately when he got my text. It made me feel so desired and idolized. And it made me feel like I was in the room with him, turning him on, even though I was on the other side of town."

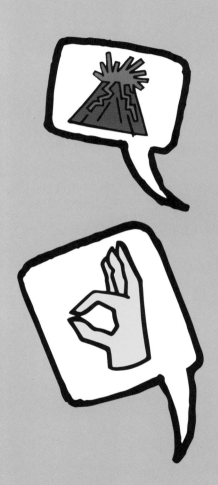

SWITCHING TENSES

Get nerdy with me about language for a moment: I swear I am not going to make you conjugate any verbs!

Anytime you're unsure of what to text, you can always talk about:

- Something you've done in the **past**
- Something you're currently doing in the **present**
- Something you want to do in the **future**

Let's say you went on a date with someone you met on OkCupid. You two had a couple of drinks after work, found you had a lot in common, and definitely decided you wanted to see each other again.

At the end of the night, as he put you in a cab, you shared a magnetic kiss. That single smooch really turned you on and had you squirming in anticipation of your next date, hopefully one involving more R-rated hanky-panky.

In a few days, you could send one of the following texts about that kiss:

Past:

> I loved the way you kissed me the other night.

In an instant, you've brought the kiss back into the forefront of his mind. Emphasizing that it was an excellent kiss makes him feel good about himself, and motivates him to give you what you want the next time you see each other.

Here is a bonus: Now he doesn't have to wonder whether it will be appropriate to lay one on you when the two of you have another date.

Present:

Right now I'm sitting at my office, but I'm dreaming of your mouth on mine.

At this very second, you are thinking about your date and that make-out session. There's a naughty thrill knowing that someone is at work, on a bus, or otherwise in public while thinking dirty thoughts—and that you are the cause of those thoughts!

Future:

The next time I see you I want to continue that amazing kiss.

Not only did you like what happened between you on that street corner, but you also want more, more, more! You are asserting what you want with confidence, while also being alluringly coy.

You can also be even more specific:

Past:

Your lips tasted delicious the other night.

. . . or more explicit:

Present:

Thinking about that kiss is making my pussy juice drip down my leg right now.

. . . or more demanding:

Future:

I want to see you Friday, and I want you to kiss me like that without any clothes on.

The past/present/future statement is an absolutely foolproof dirty talk technique, in person or over text. There's a reason "What are you wearing right now?" is the most classic phone sex trope. It persists, despite cliché, because of the immediacy of the description.

GREAT P/P/F SEXTS

Past: Devilish praise for what has happened

You fucked me so hard last night I could barely sit down this morning.

Holy shit. How many times did I cum this weekend? I seriously lost count.

Mmmmm . . . you looked so fucking hot while you were pounding me.

Present: Racy narration of what is happening

I'm in your bed and I can smell you all over me.

I just got out of the shower and I'm feeling so warm and ready for you.

I'm wearing those green panties you like.

Future: Playful threats of what's going to happen

Oh my god, baby, I cannot wait to get my hands on you tomorrow.

I hope you're well rested because you're not getting any sleep tonight.

Goddammit, I need to feel you on top of me as soon as possible.

FLIRTING TEXTS VERSUS TEXT SEX

Let's get back to those two different types of sexts we talked about. You may be in an everyday fully clothed scenario while exchanging raunchy messages: the purpose of this communication is a kind of intellectual supplement to your sex life. "Text sex" is a little bit more involved. It's the modern version of phone sex, where your texts provide the stimulation for your masturbating partner.

It may help to think of flirting texts as a light feathery touch on someone's neck and text sex as a powerful vibrator right on someone's clit.

It is, of course, quite challenging to pleasure oneself while simultaneously typing, which explains why so many website message board comments contain such horrible syntax. Even if you were to, say, insert a butt plug or put a hands-free vibrator in your underwear, it's still really, um, hard to concentrate on typing when you're getting really turned on. This is obviously part of the fun. When your partner's texts become more and more monosyllabic you know you're having that desired flustering effect.

You can describe what you're doing, or spin a complete fantasy. You're providing a sexual service, in the same way you might give a blow job to please your partner. Just like with a blow job, you may enjoy making someone else come and not necessarily need everything to be reciprocated immediately. However, if someone always expects you to provide erotic stimulation, you need to demand that your needs also be met.

GETTING PLENTY OF MILEAGE

There is no law of diminishing returns for our favorite filthy language. When you discover a word or sentence or fantasy that works, don't hesitate to use it again and again, like a catchphrase. If you like using a particular word in bed, chances are you'll like seeing it typed out over and over.

Text sex is more likely to be explicit and repetitive, almost like an incantation. Your words can become as stimulating as a body or toy. This is most likely to be in the present tense, as in:

I'm reaching my hands into my underwear now.

Oh my god, I'm so wet for you!

I'm teasing my clit and playing with my nipples.

Mmmm, my nipples are getting hard now. I wish you were here to lick them.

I'm dipping my fingers into my pussy and getting my fingers wet . . .

Please let me cum for you . . . ooh god, I'm cumming!

Oh my god, babe, that was fucking amazing, I came so hard.

DON'T BE LAZY! USE ACRONYMS SPARINGLY

omg I'm so excited for our date lol

text me l8r, k? brb

u there?

wtf

Since it takes more time to type than talk, we've invented a whole bunch of abbreviations in order to text faster. Acronyms such as WTF have entered the lexicon with such strength that you'll often hear "Double-you-tee-eff" or "Oh-em-gee!" out loud even though they have *more* syllables than the original phrase does.

You don't have to worry about coming off like a preadolescent if you type OMFG over and over again in response to sexts, as long as you realize you're using it for emphasis and not just as a place-holder. If you overuse abbreviations such as LOL, you end up sounding as if you're constantly nervously laughing, like someone who is really tense on a first date.

And feel free to sign off with XO if you really are sending hugs and kisses.

GRAMMAR AND PUNCTUATION

Now I am giving you permission to use text slang, but you have to do something for me in return. Please use good grammar and type in complete sentences, or at least use fragments that make sense. If you wouldn't say it out loud, don't type it.

As for punctuation, I wholeheartedly endorse the use of multiple exclamation marks, but only if you really want to emphasize that you are super excited.

The person who overuses exclamation points is sort of the grammatical equivalent of the boy who cried wolf. When you actually want to make a point it doesn't come across! Because it seems like you are constantly shouting!

As for periods, I don't think they are entirely necessary unless you are typing several sentences per text. In general, breaking a message up into several texts has the effect of a line break, which sort of turns your texting into poetry.

last night was amazing

omfg

*

I'm dripping down my leg

oh yeah?

I can't stop thinking about your naked body

So what are you doing for your lunch break?

Nothing...

Wanna come over and get fucked?

Be right there!

See how the anticipation is built by the following sexts, thinking of each line as its own message:

> I want

> to cum

> all over

> your cock

> tonight

> I want

> to

> soak

> your

> sheets

Try saying each of the following versions out loud based on punctuation and spelling cues, to understand how they come across conversationally.

> I want you

> i want you

> I want you.

> I want you so bad

> I want you

> So bad

> I want you so bad!

> I want you! So bad!

> I want you soooooooooooo BAD!!

GREAT DIRTY TALK
AND SEXTING IN POP CULTURE

SONGS

"How Many Licks" by Lil' Kim

"Blow" by Beyoncé

"Oops (Oh My)" by Tweet and Missy "Misdemeanor" Elliott

"I Want Your Sex" by George Michael

"I Just Wanna Make Love to You" by Etta James

"Ignition (Remix)" by R. Kelly

"Darling Nikki," "Head," "Jack U Off," "Do Me, Baby," "Cream," or basically anything by Prince

"I Need a Little Sugar in My Bowl" by Bessie Smith

"Je T'Aime Moi Non Plus" by Serge Gainsbourg and Jane Birkin

"Sexx Laws" by Beck

"Close the Door" by Teddy Pendergrass

"Justify My Love" by Madonna

"He Was a Big Freak" by Betty Davis

MOVIES

Her

The Truth about Cats and Dogs

Get Carter

Last Tango in Paris

Wild at Heart

Baby Boy

Y Tu Mamá También

Girl 6

Secretary

A WORD ON EMOJI

Emoji are the colorful little icons that come with most smartphones. They're experiencing a bit of a zeitgeist at the moment (I just saw a minidress in a store window emblazoned with High-Five Hands and Heart-Eyed Smiley Faces). Some people consider them juvenile, but my pervy friends and I are staunchly pro-Emoji.

Often those charming symbols improve on superficial small talk and can sometimes become a secret code among friends and lovers. Most important, an Emoji of the Peach That Looks Like a Butt next to the Hovering Hand That Looks Like It's Mid-Spank never fails to make me smile (see number 4 in my "Top Ten Dirty Emoji Phrases").

Emoji function like any other form of communication. When you are first getting to know someone, it's best to stick to generally understood symbols,

like Happy Face or Sparkly Heart. This can bring a little taste of your personality and communication style into texting better than mere words.

When someone sends me a Thumbs Up, I tend to imagine that person smiling and giving me the approving gesture, whereas if he typed "ok" I would think of him being sort of grouchy.

When you get to know someone better, you may start to develop an Emoji dialect that makes you both giggle. Since they're generally positive symbols, they're perfect for expressing sincerity, silliness, or just not taking yourself too seriously.

TOP TEN DIRTY EMOJI PHRASES

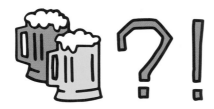

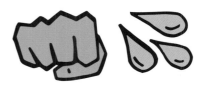

1. Let's go to the bar tonight?

2. I want to fist you until you squirt.

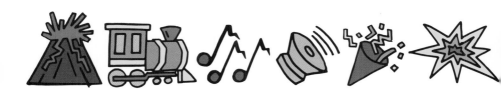

3. You make me cum so hard.

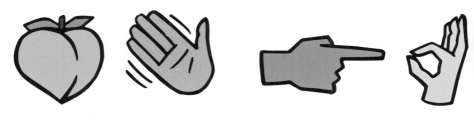

4. Spank me.

5. Let's fuck.

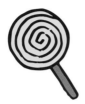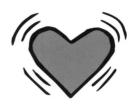

6. I wanna lick you.

7. You make me gush.

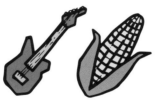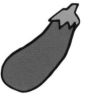

8. You make me hard.

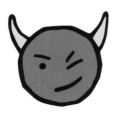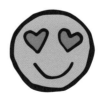

9. I'm horny.

10. I've got a crush on you.

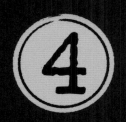

SEND SEXY PICTURES AND VIDEO:
A Selfie Says a Thousand (Dirty) Words

Everybody knows that pornography drives technology. Whether it's the printing press or VHS, photography or streaming video, the first thing that humans want to do with a new advancement in communication is share hardcore content.

We are now living in a golden age of digital possibilities, where most of us have access to personalized smut-making machines. For this reason, "porn" doesn't just mean commercial sexual media anymore. Porn can also be any picture or video you create and share with a special someone in order to tease, turn on, seduce, and stay connected.

This section will give you all the tools you need to make sexy stills and movies in seconds. Whether you're taking selfies that will make your mate blush or choosing the flattering avatar picture that expresses the real you, these tips will get you prepped to become a sexual supermodel.

I've also provided guidelines for putting on an erotic Skype show, so you can feel right in the room with your long-distance lover. Or, if your boo is just across town, you'll learn how to create a sexy Snapchat that will disappear as soon as it has been watched.

Of course, these pictures should only be for you and the people you trust. I'll also give guidelines for protecting your privacy so you can show off unafraid and unashamed.

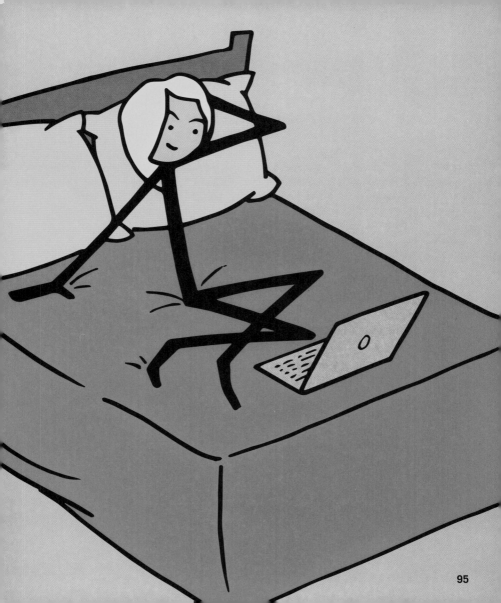

CHOOSING PROFILE PICTURES

Critics tend to bemoan the rise of hookup apps such as Tinder and Grindr, claiming we are becoming a world of superficial daters. You shouldn't feel guilty about the fact that visual attraction is a key component of your search for a good match.

Be Here Now: Make sure the picture is updated and reflects what you look like nowadays. If you, like me, change your hair color constantly, just make sure you have at least one casual snapshot that shows your new 'do.

Make Eye Contact with the Camera: Look at a series of advertisements and ask yourself: Do you feel more connected to the models who fix the camera with a stone-cold gaze or the ones who stare blankly off into the distance? Chances are, you like the ones who seem to be looking into your soul.

Illuminate Yourself: As any professional photographer will tell you, lighting is *everything*. Diffused lighting is always the most flattering, which means outdoor shots are ideal and flash is the enemy. Shoot for a happy medium between too posed (which can come across as aloof) and too amateur (glowing red eyes won't do you any favors). Don't use so many filters that you look alien or blown out. Under no circumstances should you use Photoshop.

Show Off Those Pearly Whites: I do not love pictures of myself smiling. Ever since I was an angsty teen, I have thought that pictures of my smiling face looked distorted and weird. But other people see the emotion expressed on my face, rather than a collection of features or perceived flaws. Choose a picture in which you were genuinely happy; it will send the message that you can make the right person happy, too.

Be Very Discerning about Choosing Pictures That Feature Other People:
Showing pictures that feature other people sends the message that you're social and outgoing, perhaps even loyal and considerate of others. These are all attractive qualities. On the other hand, I tend to find these pictures confusing. Even if you indicate which one is you, I find myself distracted by the other people, especially if they're also cute! Ideally, the picture with friends should clearly *feature* you.

Profile pictures of you with others are okay, but make sure you are clearly featured to avoid confusion.

Include Some Action Shots: If you really love to do something, chances are your friends have snapped a candid picture of you doing it.

Use that photo of your sweaty face twisted in concentration as your foot collides with a soccer ball. Check the Facebook wall of your favorite dance party for one perfect shot of your makeup-smeared face getting down to your favorite Rihanna track. If you have a picture of yourself playing the guitar onstage, live action role-playing in the park, or making sushi for a dinner party, throw it up there!

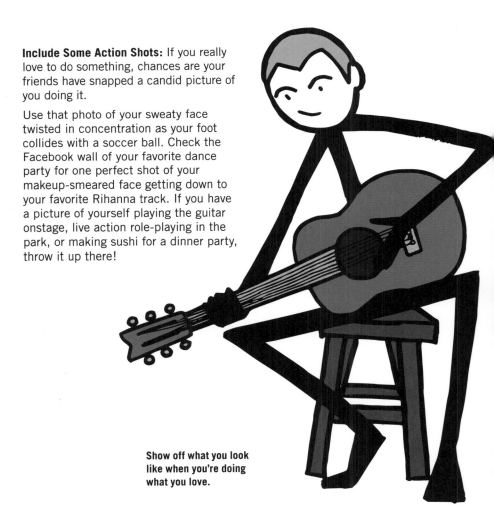

Show off what you look like when you're doing what you love.

Picking the Right One: Narrow it down to ten choices and show them to a friend. The ideal friend judge is attracted to your gender and will be encouraging yet honest.

Judging Profiles Based on Pictures: To figure out how to judge the profiles of others based on pictures, simply reverse the above rules! You want to set your sights on someone who isn't afraid to smile, who has passionate interests, and who knows how to use a freaking digital camera.

IF YOU HAVE TO CHOOSE FIVE PICTURES, TRY ONE IN EACH OF THE FOLLOWING CATEGORIES

Emotion: smiling, having fun, candid, relaxed

Body: full-body shot, eye contact, sexy and smoldering

Action: enjoying something you love

Face: posed or professional shot, if you have one, or your best selfie

Friends: group shot with you at the center

IN DEFENSE OF THE SELFIE

The modern culture of selfie taking catches a lot of flak. "We have become a society of egomaniacs," quoth the cynics, "each citizen a Narcissus obsessively staring into the shallow pool of his or her own reflection."

To this I say: Whatever, fellas. We woke up like this.

Most critiques of vanity are inherently based on sexist double standards, by which women (and gay men) are expected to be perfect objects of masculine desire while never appearing to be trying too hard. Practiced in moderation, the act of admiring yourself and expecting idolization from others is perfectly healthy for your self-esteem.

More relevant to our purposes here, selfies show that you're sexy and you know it, and that confidence is very attractive.

Another reason that selfies are kind of revolutionary is that they cut out the middleman and restore agency to the subject of the picture: a.k.a. the model, a.k.a. *you*. You don't need to rely on someone else to take the perfectly angled portrait of your visage, or show off your body the way you want to be admired. A selfie proclaims, "You now have to see me the way I see myself."

GREAT REASONS TO SEND A SEXY SELFIE

1. To give your partner something personalized to masturbate to
2. To show off and feel sexy
3. To flirt and encourage someone to come over
4. To seduce and let someone know what you want later
5. To show attention, affection, and love
6. Because it turns you on and/or turns your partner on
7. Because it shows trust
8. Because it will motivate your partner to send one back
9. Because it's silly and fun
10. Because your partner is having a lousy day and you want to alleviate stress

SELFIE SELF-LOVE

Sometimes a sexy picture doesn't have to be for someone else: it can just be for you! I love taking pictures of myself when I look killer and feel on top of the world. I'll flip through these shots when I'm not feeling so hot about myself. It puts me in a better mood to be reminded of a moment when I was feeling positive about my body.

Then, of course, one of the great pleasures of taking a juicy picture is sending it to someone you know will appreciate it. There are different kinds of attention you might want to solicit. You can absolutely send a hot picture of yourself to a good friend to get the affirmation that you look amazing. This can also normalize your exhibitionism and help you feel bold enough to send it to a date.

HOW TO BE REALLY GOOD
AT RECEIVING NAKED PICTURES

When your inbox lights up with a sexy photo, be gracious and grateful! Even if you don't know what to say back, even if you think the picture is over-the-top and silly, show your gratitude.

A friend recently told me that no matter how passionately she texted "I wanna suck your cock tonight," to her boyfriend with an alluring picture of her red lipstick–painted open mouth, she could never get more than a monosyllabic reply. Perhaps her boyfriend considered it unmanly to respond with enthusiasm, but he was incorrect. Nobody is going to keep sending you sexy photos if all you give back is "nice."

If you are saving sexy pictures on your phone, lock and password protect them. You are now responsible for the privacy of your date's naked pictures as well as your own stash. There are smartphone apps that act as storage vaults and password protect your private nudes.

It should go without saying: Don't be a creep. Never, *ever* forward a picture meant for you to anyone else. Don't post it on a website and don't print it out. Don't even let someone glance at it over your shoulder. Show that you are worthy of trust and deserving of the delicious photos you've received.

ASK FIRST

A good way to solicit a sexy picture is to send one first. The only way to make certain someone wants to see a sexy picture of you is to ask first:

> I'm really hard for you right now and I want to show you.

> I just got home from the gym and I'm really sweaty, wanna see?

The failsafe response to a sexy picture is a sexy picture of you! If you get a shot of a mouth, respond with your mouth. If you get a teasing half-naked shot, respond in kind.

If you're hoping to see a little bit more, up the ante yourself. Lift up your shirt and pull down your pants slightly, perhaps revealing a peek of pubic hair. The idea is to mirror your partner while coaxing things a little further. It's very exciting to receive a picture knowing your partner sees what you're getting at.

Remember, don't send a picture of your genitals unless someone asks for it. It's really that simple.

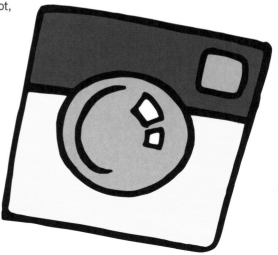

HOW TO TAKE A GREAT SEXY SELFIE

Did I mention eye contact? Gaze through the camera as though someone you want to fuck is on the other side.

Don't get lost in the dark. Make sure you use good lighting so the recipient can see what you're sending.

Shoot from above. This helps emphasize your eyes and avoid double chins.

Shoot from below. Accentuate the shape of your chest, butt, or crotch.

PYT POV. For your pretty young thing point of view, lie on your back. Hold the camera above your head as if your partner were inside the camera, looking down on you. Or place the camera in any other position you want your partner to be in, like between your legs looking up at you.

Use great reference material. Look at some great hardcore porn or images from fashion magazines. Notice how many of the positions they use over and over are flattering and erotic regardless of body type.

Get yourself really turned on. Let your horniness show in the picture. Open your mouth, writhe around on your back, and get sweaty!

Touch yourself! Run your hands all over your face, your chest, your ass, and your junk. Tweak your nipples. Suck on your finger. Ever notice how a pop star like Katy Perry runs her hands all over herself during performances? It sends this message: Right now *I'm* touching me, but *you* could be touching me!

Skip the selfie. Use your camera's built-in timer and simple tripod. Better yet, ask a friend to do you a favor and play photographer. A good friend will also be honest with you about your most flattering angles.

Get more control. Cradling your phone in your hand, click the button on the side of your phone instead of contorting yourself to hit the front button.

Don't end up on SelfieswithBoredCats. Tumblr.com. Make sure your image dominates the picture and there's nothing distracting in it that would take away from the focus on you.

Go through a glass darkly. Shoot your reflection in the mirror. Definitely turn the flash off. The most popular mirror pose is with the phone in the middle of the chest, but I'm also a fan of holding the phone up and off to the side. You can either look at the camera or look into the mirror, although it can be challenging to make sure your gaze looks natural.

Go forth and multiply! To get fancy, angle your mirror picture so that it shows your face and backside simultaneously.

The butt selfie. Hold the camera out as far as you can, twist your spine, and angle it from below to show off your curves.

The reclining bikini POV. Celebrities use this one a lot on Instagram, but you don't have to be in Ibiza to get the effect. Hold the camera close to your face and frame your chest in the foreground with your toes twinkling on the horizon. This elongates your body and distinctly demonstrates that you're admiring yourself.

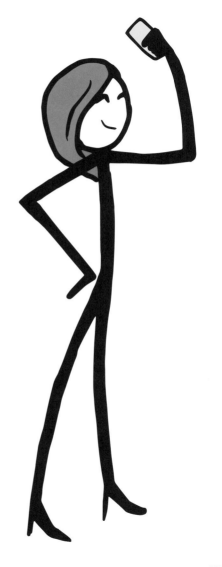

The number one rule for a sexy selfie: make eye contact!

WHY IS SNAPCHAT SO GREAT?

Snapchat is an app that allows you to send pictures and short videos to other users. Its novel appeal is that, unlike pretty much anything else you send, snaps disappear after they are viewed. The impermanence has obvious appeal for privacy, but it also creates an exciting sense of concentration and urgency. You can also caption your snap, combining lewd images with indecent proposals.

Just beware that the recipient of your snap can take a screenshot, making the photo not-so-temporary.

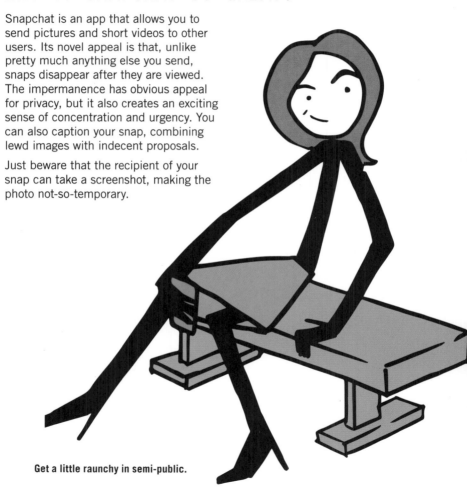

Get a little raunchy in semi-public.

IDEAS FOR SNAPCHATS

The Tease

Hold your phone between your legs and film a close-up of your fingers gently stroking yourself.

Make sexy noises in the background—moans, gasps, or X-rated utterances.

Hot caption: *"This is what I want your tongue to do to me," "This is what I like to do to myself when you're not here," "I want to cum on your cock."*

The Bounce

Focus on a sexy part of your body, like your breasts or ass, then grope, jiggle, or undulate for the camera.

The Rocky Horror

Close up on your mouth saying something seductive like, *"I want you in my mouth tonight."* Slowly lick your lips.

The Penetrating Gaze

Look deep into the camera as if your partner were right on the other side.

The Kinky Suggestion

Show off something kinky that turns you on, like slapping your own ass with a wooden hairbrush, licking a leather boot, or putting clothespins on your nipples.

Hot caption: *"I've been very bad, Daddy."*

The Show-Off

Put your hands down your pants or up your skirt in a semi-public area, like a restaurant bathroom or an empty train car.

The Poly Advantage

If you're nonmonogamous, film yourself kissing someone cute and send it to your date.

Hot caption: *"Now it's your turn."*

The Double Entendre

Shoot a close-up of your tongue licking an ice cream cone or wrapping your lips around a Popsicle.

Hot caption: *"I need your sugar in my mouth."*

The Temptation

Pan over your entire naked body.

Hot caption: *"This can be yours if you wanna come over."*

The Fashionista

Show off the impeccable outfit you're wearing for your date tonight.

SENDING AND RECEIVING SEXY VIDEOS

When I started directing porn, I knew next to nothing about filmmaking. It was 2009, and all I had was a Flip cam, which at the time was a cutting-edge mini camcorder about the size and quality of a smartphone.

Being a pornographer was a very forgiving way to learn filmmaking. If the sound was bad, but the sex was hot, it was good porn. If the continuity was lousy, but the sex was hot, it was good porn.

This is true of taking sexy pictures and videos of yourself as well. You don't have to be Sofia Coppola to create something that captures the mood, movement, and personality of your desire.

IDEAS FOR EXCITING SEX TAPES

These clips can be thirty seconds or two hours long. They can be shared privately or uploaded to an amateur porn site for an extra exhibitionist thrill. You can send the video to your boo to tease him about an upcoming rendezvous, or to remind her how much she wants to be close to you when you're far away.

The Reveal

Pull your underwear to one side and show 'em what you're workin' with.

When I Think About You I Touch Myself

Enjoy your alone time! You can even pretend the camera isn't there, or treat the camera like a character that you are teasing.

Be theatrical! Use props and costumes! Dildos, vibrators, butt plugs, strap-on harnesses, lingerie, leather boots, stockings, and garter belt—whatever appeals to your and your partner's tastes.

Be Your Own Voyeur

When you and your partner are together, set up your camera next to the bed and film your sex.

Later you can masturbate to yourself!

Send the video to your partner when you're far away to remind him what he's missing.

What's Your Fantasy?

Act out a scene or character from a TV show or comic book you both like.

This can be playful or extremely detail-oriented, depending on what tickles your fancy.

Cut to the Chase

Work yourself up and switch on the camera at the moment of orgasm.

Aural Fixation

Skip the visuals and take advantage of racy sound effects.

Make a voice memo of yourself masturbating. The sound of your moans and screams are sure to arouse your partner in a surprising way. Plus, she can listen to it on her headphones in public without anyone knowing.

Instant Porn Star

Make a video of yourself masturbating. Prop your phone up against a book, or buy a simple tripod stand to hold it in place. Then upload it to an amateur porn site and send your partner the link.

Make amateur porn together and post it online with mutual consent. Enjoy the exhibitionist thrill of watching yourself in virtual public, and the idea that other people are watching and getting off to your sex life.

Obey this cardinal rule:
DO NOT READ THE COMMENTS.

LIVE SEX SHOW: VIDEOCHAT

What is it about video chatting that makes it seem like I'm living in the future? There's something kind of surreal about feeling mentally and visually really close to someone who is physically far away.

Video chatting helps you feel close to your partner when you can't be in the same room. Whether you're in a long-distance relationship, getting through a period of temporary travel, or just living on the other side of town, video chatting helps you stay sexy even on nights that aren't date nights.

WHY IS SKYPE SEX SO HOT?

1. You're giving each other masturbation fodder, which is a generous and loving act.

2. You can enjoy simultaneous exhibitionism and voyeurism with one person from the comfort of your own private room.

3. You can view close-ups of parts of your partner that you don't see during sex.

4. You learn how your partner gets off alone.

5. The physical distance can inspire you to get creative and adventurous.

6. Because you can't physically stimulate each other, you're encouraged to dirty talk, to say what you like about sex and what you fantasize about.

7. You're essentially directing customized porn in real time.

8. You can watch yourself from your partner's perspective. Or you can choose to turn that screen off and focus on your partner.

9. You can take screenshots to enjoy later.

10. You can tease your partner and inspire each other's yearning to be close again.

SOME GREAT SKYPE/FACETIME IDEAS

Spread It

Lie on your back, place the computer between your legs, prop your back up on a pillow, and run your fingers all over yourself. If you're feeling too shy to watch the screen, stare up at the ceiling and listen to your partner describe how gorgeous you are.

Git Along Little Doggie

Turn around and get on all fours, showing your butt off for your partner—this is another great one if you're feeling too shy to look.

Undulate and arch your back as if you're doing cat and cow yoga poses.

Twerk it!

Toy Story

Give head to a dildo or finger.

No need to deep throat unless that's your pleasure—just show lots of tongue and pouty lips.

Take Turns

Switch off being a masturbation voyeur and an exhibitionist.

Switch off being dominant and submissive, instructing each other in what you want to see.

Have an Entire Date

Stare at each other, breathe away the nervousness, giggle, and talk.

Let the sexy times develop naturally, as they would in person.

Afterward, pull the computer up close for some remote pillow talk.

KEEPING YOUR PARTS PRIVATE

Just because you chose to create and share images of your naked body doesn't mean you need to live in fear of humiliating exposure. Digital security is a serious concern, and even exhibitionists have a right to privacy.

ME? A PORN STAR?

Twentieth-century men's magazines perpetuated a particular kind of ideal beauty. You know the type—the Barbie with the flat stomach, perky (or augmented) breasts, long sleek legs, and agreeable bimbo attitude. This isn't necessarily what *most* people find attractive. It just happens to be *Playboy* mogul Hugh Hefner's type, and for a long time Hugh was the powerful man who paid the bills.

As a result, many of us learn that we have to look a certain way in order to show off our bodies. This simply isn't true. Everyone is beautiful, and there is always someone out there who thinks you're beautiful. Remember, part of the appeal of the naked person in a picture is the way she shows off her vulnerability and her particular expression of sexiness.

Counterintuitively, we also blame and shame women who show off their bodies proudly. Women must always look presentable but never betray their effort. Look no further for proof of this double standard than the ongoing controversies over the hacking of celebrities' private photos. Countless famous actresses, including Scarlett Johansson and Jennifer Lawrence, have had to address backlash after their private nude pictures were stolen and uploaded onto the Internet for anyone to see. Many conservative critiques of these crimes have chastised these women for taking naked photos in the first place. By this reasoning, these women deserved to have their pictures viewed by the world, because they were irresponsible enough to take them. This is complete bullshit.

All adults have a right to their own sexual expression. We need to respect one another's agency in using modern tools to explore, experiment, and share our sexuality. There is absolutely nothing wrong with taking naked pictures of yourself or with the mutually consensual sharing of hardcore images.

Remember, there are people in this world who choose to publicize titillating images of themselves, who profit off these images or are in control of the rights. Unfortunately, despite a proliferation of sex workers producing and selling erotic entertainment, people do seem to enjoy the thrill of looking at something they know they aren't supposed to see—that is, stolen nude pictures. It's unethical to post or view pictures that are nonconsensually shared, not to pose for those pictures in private.

We should all consider risks and consequences in our sexual adventures. Just as the only 100 percent effective form of birth control is abstinence, the only way to be completely assured that your fabulous butt selfie will not end up on FabulousButtSelfies.tumblr.com is, sadly, not to take fabulous butt selfies. If you cannot handle the idea of not having control of your naked pictures, then don't take them or send them.

As we all know, people make informed risks every day and have incredible sex lives without ever having an unwanted pregnancy. You could sext to your heart's content and never experience a violation of trust. It's all part of the excitement and responsibility of being a sexually active grown-up.

STRATEGIES FOR KEEPING CONTENT PRIVATE

1. Store all your nude and hardcore pictures in a special folder or use a storage site or application.

2. Take the time to secure your email and storage with passcodes that aren't full words and security questions that aren't easy for others to guess.

3. Only share your pictures with people you really trust.

4. If someone tries to share his girlfriend's nude picture with you, tell him you don't want to see it (even/ especially if you really, really do!). Remind him this is a violation of trust, or simply say, "I only like naked pictures of girls who consent to me seeing them naked."

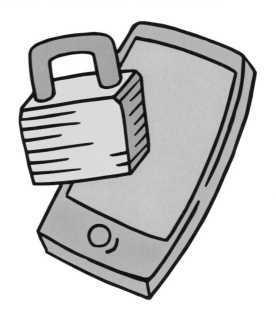

Got nudes on your phone? Lock 'em up.

STRATEGIES FOR PROTECTING YOUR ANONYMITY

Although you should never be ashamed to flaunt what you got, it's also important to recognize that an image of you has a life of its own. Here are some ways to minimize risks of unwanted exposure while still enjoying the life of a show-off.

Face/Off

Shoot yourself in a way that doesn't show your face or any distinguishing marks, such as tattoos.

Hold the phone in front of your face while taking a mirror selfie.

The pure self-objectification inherent to a picture of your body sans face has its own erotic charge.

Ready for My Close-Up

Shoot extreme close-ups between your legs, of your chest, butt, or mouth.

Close-ups of the body can make ordinary anatomy into something surreally gorgeous. One unexpected thing about these pictures is that sometimes sex is so stimulating we don't have time to focus in on any one thing. Or it's improbable to be able to see, for example, what a penis looks like going in and out of a vagina.

Conceal Yourself with a Costume

If you do have tattoos, wear sexy clothes or blankets that cover them.

Some people find partially clothed bodies even sexier than nude bodies, especially if they have a fetish for items like corsets or stockings.

Your idea of what constitutes "sexy clothes" may vary. An old band T-shirt and boxers could be just as alluring as a satin teddy.

Go Undercover

Wear a leather blindfold or a corny masquerade mask.

Anything that covers part of your face evokes a certain mystery.

Instant Fetish Star

If you want more complete anonymity, indulge in a full-head hood.

Hoods come in leather, latex, or more affordable synthetic materials. Some look like bunnies or piggies, if that gets you going.

Hoods can be incredibly sexy for sensory deprivation and can be a great way to explore how it feels to wear fetish gear.

Be Suggestive

Cum all over the bed and take a picture of the soaked sheets (hint: put a coin next to the puddle for scale).

Take a picture of your favorite dildo or lingerie on the bed, a box of condoms or gloves, or a brand-new bottle of lube.

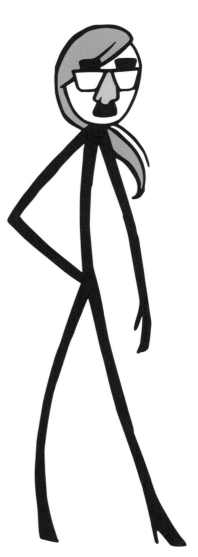

A FINAL WORD ON PRIVACY

A lot of the hand-wringing over nude selfies and amateur porn has to do with the perceived threat of blackmail or humiliation if these photos are leaked. The criminals who steal images, or petty exes who post them, would have no power if a naked picture of you weren't inherently humiliating.

Maybe what we all really need to do is adjust our feelings about what it means to be exposed. Think about it—instead of living in fear that someone will see you naked, maybe try not to care who sees you naked. If your nakedness is a source of pride and power instead of furtive secrecy, then no one can use your pictures to hurt you!

Aren't we all just looking for someone to spoon with?

IN CONCLUSION

With the rise of social media and online dating, we begin to hear some common questions: Are we devaluing each person we date because we have the power of possibilities buzzing in our pockets? Do we increasingly expect obscene digital gifts from one another at the expense of decreased intimacy and compassion? When you walk into a bar and see denizens hunched over their devices, faces illuminated by a pale blue light, a dystopia of alienation starts to feel eerily plausible.

Maybe it's naïve, but I truly believe that our drive to connect and belong will override the most monolithic of technological advancements. Sometimes people hide behind machines, and sometimes they use their anonymity as an excuse to act careless, inconsiderate, or even abusive. Yet I cannot tell you how many people I have met who thought they were utterly alone . . . until the Internet helped them connect with other people who shared their desires.

My vision of the future of sexual technology is that we will learn how to use the machines to communicate better, to generate pleasure and understanding. People want to take risks and break each other's hearts. We want it all: to be cruel and kind and selfish and giving. We want to be surprised by sensation. We want to make someone's day better, to feel pride in making a partner scream in orgasm. We want to play and jump on the bed and make each other laugh and wake up spooning each other.

We want the things that can never be done virtually. No matter how much we become conditioned by innovative tools, we will continue to be drawn to the scent of each other's sweat and the thumping of one another's hearts.

ACKNOWLEDGMENTS

Thanks to Sarah, Lisa, Ryan, and Andie for your insightful notes.

Thanks to Quinn Cassidy, Maggie Mayhem, Andre Shakti, and Casey Grey, for dirty talking professionally with me for all these years.

Thanks to Cassandra Seale for putting in a good word for me!

I am indebted to the writers and teachers who have smack-talked their way into my world: Tristan Taormino, Carol Queen, Diana Cage, Laura Antoniou, Patrick Califia, Melissa Gira Grant, Siouxsie Q, Audacia Ray, Sinclair Sexsmith, Lorelei Lee, Barbara Carrellas, Reid Mihalko, Douglas Rushkoff, Julia Serano, Ignacio Rivera, Randall Kenan, and Samuel R. Delany.

Thank you to the venues who booked my Dirty Talk workshops, allowing me to develop the principals that informed this book, among them Good Vibrations, Good For Her, Kink Academy, the San Francisco Citadel, Sharrin Spector and Pat Baillie at International Ms Leather, the Lesbian Sex Mafia, MOBB, and Armory Studios. Thanks to everyone who ever attended one of those workshops and had the nerve to scream the word *cunt!* in a room full of strangers.

Thanks to Jennifer Pritchett and Smitten Kitten for underwriting my podcast *Why Are People Into That?!* and supporting our communities.

Thanks to Jessica Haberman for being everything an editor should be: precise, respectful, anecdotal, and hilarious. And thanks to Cara Connors and the Fair Winds team.

To my sweet bear: I really get a dirty mind whenever you're around.

This book was written to the tune of Solange's *SoL-AngeL & the Hadley Street Dreams* (Instrumental) album, *Black Messiah* by D'Angelo, *The Story of Moondog*, and a hell of a lot of Serge Gainsbourg.

Tina Horn is a writer, teacher, and media-maker. She produces and hosts the sexuality podcast *Why Are People Into That?!* Her first book, *Love Not Given Lightly*, is a collection of nonfiction stories about sex workers; she has also been published in *Vice, Nerve, Girl Sex 101*, and *Best Sex Writing 2015*. Tina's workshops on dirty talk, sex worker self-care, and spanking have been featured at Good Vibrations, Armory Studios, Lesbian Sex Mafia, International Ms Leather, and the Feminist Porn Conference. She is a LAMBDA Literary Fellow, has won two Feminist Porn Awards, and holds an MFA in creative nonfiction writing from Sarah Lawrence. Born in Northern California, Tina now lives in Manhattan. Find her at TinaHorn. net and @TinaHornsAss.

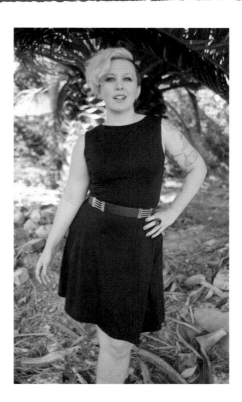

Books

Opening Up by Tristan Taormino

The Sexual Life of Catherine M by Catherine Millet

The Smart Girl's Guide to Porn by Violet Blue

Exhibitionism for the Shy by Carol Queen

Any erotica anthology edited by Rachel Kramer Bussel

The Marketplace Series by Laura Antoniou

Girl Sex 101 by Allison Moon and kd diamond

Macho Sluts by Pat Califia

Ecstasy Is Necessary by Barbara Carrellas

Blogs

Sugarbutch Chronicles, www.sugarbutch.net, by Sinclair Sexsmith

Oh Joy Sex Toy, www.ohjoysextoy.com, by Erika Moen and Matthew Nolan

Podcasts

The Whorecast

Sex Out Loud

Savage Love

Sex Coaches

Reid Mihalko

Charlie Glickman

Porn Performers Who Are Also Writers

Lorelei Lee

Conner Habib

Jiz Lee

Joanna Angel

Siouxsie Q

Maxine Holloway

DVDs

Rough Sex series
directed by Tristan Taormino

Nina Hartley's Guide to Seduction

Crash Pad Series directed by Shine
Louise Houston

*Talk To Me Baby: A Lover's Guide to Dirty
Talk and Role-Play* hosted by Shar Renoir